D0086174

Procedures Checklist

to Accompany
Foundations of Basic Nursing

Third Edition

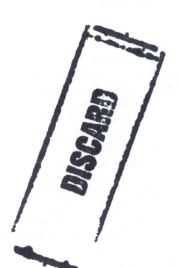

Lois White, RN, PhD
Gena Duncan, RN, MSEd, MSN
Wendy Baumle, RN, MSN

Prepared by
Shawn White, RN, BSN
Griffin Technical College
Griffin, Georgia

PAUL D. CAMP COMMUNITY COLLEGE
271 KENYON ROAD
SUFFOLK, VIRGINIA 23434

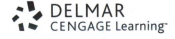

DELMAR
CENGAGE Learning™

Australia • Brazil • Japan • Korea • Mexico • Singapore • Spain • United Kingdom • United States

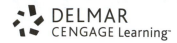
DELMAR
CENGAGE Learning™

Procedures Checklist to accompany Foundations of Basic Nursing, Third Edition

By Lois White, RN, PhD, Gena Duncan, MSEd, MSN, and Wendy Baumle, MSN

Vice President, Career and Professional Editorial: Dave Garza

Director of Learning Solutions: Matt Kane

Executive Editor: Steven Helba

Managing Editor: Marah Bellegarde

Senior Product Manager: Juliet Steiner

Editorial Assistant: Meghan E. Orvis

Vice President, Career and Professional Marketing: Jennifer Ann Baker

Executive Marketing Manager: Wendy Mapstone

Senior Marketing Manager: Michele McTighe

Marketing Coordinator: Scott Chrysler

Production Director: Carolyn Miller

Production Manager: Andrew Crouth

Senior Content Project Manager: James Zayicek

Senior Art Director: Jack Pendleton

© 2011, 2005, 2001 Delmar, Cengage Learning

ALL RIGHTS RESERVED. No part of this work covered by the copyright herein may be reproduced, transmitted, stored, or used in any form or by any means graphic, electronic, or mechanical, including but not limited to photocopying, recording, scanning, digitizing, taping, Web distribution, information networks, or information storage and retrieval systems, except as permitted under Section 107 or 108 of the 1976 United States Copyright Act, without the prior written permission of the publisher.

For product information and technology assistance, contact us at **Professional & Career Group Customer Support, 1-800-648-7450**

For permission to use material from this text or product, submit all requests online at **cengage.com/permissions**. Further permissions questions can be e-mailed to **permissionrequest@cengage.com**.

Library of Congress Control Number: 2009929886
ISBN-13: 9781428317840
ISBN-10: 1428317848

Delmar
5 Maxwell Drive
Clifton Park, NY 12065-2919
USA

Cengage Learning products are represented in Canada by Nelson Education, Ltd.

For your lifelong learning solutions, visit **delmar.cengage.com**
Visit our corporate website at **cengage.com**.

NOTICE TO THE READER

Publisher does not warrant or guarantee any of the products described herein or perform any independent analysis in connection with any of the product information contained herein. Publisher does not assume, and expressly disclaims, any obligation to obtain and include information other than that provided to it by the manufacturer. The reader is expressly warned to consider and adopt all safety precautions that might be indicated by the activities described herein and to avoid all potential hazards. By following the instructions contained herein, the reader willingly assumes all risks in connection with such instructions. The publisher makes no representations or warranties of any kind, including but not limited to, the warranties of fitness for particular purpose or merchantability, nor are any such representations implied with respect to the material set forth herein, and the publisher takes no responsibility with respect to such material. The publisher shall not be liable for any special, consequential, or exemplary damages resulting, in whole or part, from the readers' use of, or reliance upon, this material.

Printed in the United States of America
1 2 3 4 5 6 7 14 13 12 11 10

CONTENTS

Chapter 31 • Advanced Procedures

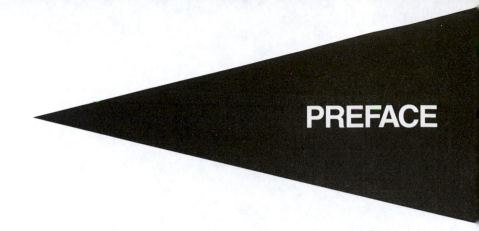

PREFACE

The skills checklists in this manual are summaries of the step-by-step procedures in the *Foundations of Nursing, Third Edition* textbook, by Lois White, Gena Duncan, and Wendy Baumle. They are arranged according to the first three steps of the nursing process:

- Assessment
- Planning/Expected Outcomes
- Implementation

Each checklist follows the procedure as described in the textbook. To use the skills checklists more effectively, the user should refer to the procedure first, then "practice," referring to the checklist.

When users are evaluated using the checklists, there are three categories to document their performances of the skills: "Able to Perform," "Able to Perform with Assistance," or "Unable to Perform." These categories lend themselves to the school laboratory setting as well as to the clinical setting, where students may perform procedures with faculty assistance.

Checklist for Procedure 29-1   Hand Hygiene

Name _____ Date _____

School _____

Instructor _____

Course _____

Procedure 29-1 Hand Hygiene	Able to Perform	Able to Perform with Assistance	Unable to Perform	Initials and Date
Assessment				
1. Assess the environment to establish if facilities are adequate for washing the hands. *Comments:*	☐	☐	☐	
2. Assess your hands to determine if they have open cuts, hangnails, broken skin, or heavily soiled areas. *Comments:*	☐	☐	☐	
3. Maintain short natural nails. Short nails harbor fewer microorganisms and do not harm clients when providing care. *Comments:*	☐	☐	☐	
Planning/Expected Outcomes				
1. The caregiver's hands are washed adequately to remove microorganisms, transient flora, and soil from the skin. *Comments:*	☐	☐	☐	
Implementation				
Handwashing 1. Remove jewelry; wristwatch may be pushed up above the wrist (midforearm). Push sleeves of uniform or shirt up above the wrist at midforearm level. *Comments:*	☐	☐	☐	
2. Assess hands for hangnails, cuts or breaks in the skin, and areas that are heavily soiled. *Comments:*	☐	☐	☐	
3. Turn on the water. Adjust the flow and temperature. The temperature of the water should be warm. *Comments:*	☐	☐	☐	
4. Wet hands and lower forearms thoroughly by holding under running water. Keep hands and forearms in the down position, with elbows straight. Avoid splashing water and touching the sides of the sink or faucet. *Comments:*	☐	☐	☐	

continued on the following page

continued from the previous page

Procedure 29-1	Able to Perform	Able to Perform with Assistance	Unable to Perform	Initials and Date
5. Apply about 5 mL (1 teaspoon) of liquid soap. Lather thoroughly. *Comments:*	☐	☐	☐	
6. Thoroughly rub hands together for about 10–15 seconds. Interlace fingers and thumbs and move back and forth to wash between digits. Wash palms, backs of hands, and wrists with firm rubbing and circular motions. Special attention should be provided to areas such as the knuckles and fingernails, which are known to harbor organisms. *Comments:*	☐	☐	☐	
7. Rinse with hands in the down position, elbows straight. Rinse in the direction of forearm to wrist to fingers. *Comments:*	☐	☐	☐	
8. Blot hands and forearms to dry thoroughly. Dry in the direction of fingers to wrist and forearms. Discard the paper towels in the proper receptacle. *Comments:*	☐	☐	☐	
9. Turn off the water faucet with a clean, dry paper towel. *Comments:*	☐	☐	☐	
Alcohol-Based Hand Rub				
10. Apply the manufacturer's recommended amount of product to one hand. *Comments:*	☐	☐	☐	
11. Rub hands together, covering hands and fingers on all sides. *Comments:*	☐	☐	☐	
12. Continue rubbing until hands are dry. *Comments:*	☐	☐	☐	
Evaluation				
1. The hand hygiene was adequate to control topical flora and infectious agents on the hands. *Comments:*	☐	☐	☐	
2. The hands were not recontaminated during or shortly after the hand hygiene. *Comments:*	☐	☐	☐	

Checklist for Procedure 29-2   Use of Protective Equipment

Name _____ Date _____

School _____

Instructor _____

Course _____

Procedure 29-2 Use of Protective Equipment	Able to Perform	Able to Perform with Assistance	Unable to Perform	Initials and Date
Assessment				
1. Assess if Standard Precautions are followed or if specific isolation precautions are needed for the client's condition. The type of microorganism and mode of transmission determine the degree of precautions. *Comments:*	☐	☐	☐	
2. Assess the client's laboratory results to learn which organism the client is infected with and the client's immune responses. *Comments:*	☐	☐	☐	
3. Assess what nursing measures are required before entering the room to have all the necessary equipment ready. *Comments:*	☐	☐	☐	
4. Assess the client's knowledge for the need to wear a cap, gown, and mask during care to direct client teaching. *Comments:*	☐	☐	☐	
5. Assess whether the isolation is airborne, droplet, or contact and which isolation attire is necessary. *Comments:*	☐	☐	☐	
Planning/Expected Outcomes				
1. The client and staff will remain free of nosocomial infection. *Comments:*	☐	☐	☐	
2. The health care provider will be protected from infection when caring for the client. *Comments:*	☐	☐	☐	
3. The staff will avoid transmitting microorganisms to others. *Comments:*	☐	☐	☐	

continued on the following page

continued from the previous page

Procedure 29-2	Able to Perform	Able to Perform with Assistance	Unable to Perform	Initials and Date
4. The client will interact on a social level with nurse, family members, and other visitors. *Comments:*	☐	☐	☐	
Implementation				
1. Wash hands. Check client's identification band. Explain procedure before beginning. *Comments:*	☐	☐	☐	
2. First put on the cap or surgical hat/hood. Hair should be tucked in a manner so that all hair is covered. *Comments:*	☐	☐	☐	
3. Apply a mask around mouth and nose and secure in a manner that prevents venting. *Comments:*	☐	☐	☐	
4. Open gown, slip arms into sleeves, and secure at neck and side. *Comments:*	☐	☐	☐	
5. Protective eyewear is worn whenever health care provider and client are at risk for splash and contamination. *Comments:*	☐	☐	☐	
6. Don clean gloves. If sterile gloves are required for a procedure, use open or closed method. *Comments:*	☐	☐	☐	
7. Use open glove technique for sterile procedures (not scrubbed). *Comments:*	☐	☐	☐	
8. Use closed glove technique if scrubbed for operating room. *Comments:*	☐	☐	☐	
9. Enter the client's room and explain the rationale for wearing the attire. *Comments:*	☐	☐	☐	

Procedure 29-2	Able to Perform	Able to Perform with Assistance	Unable to Perform	Initials and Date
10. After performing necessary tasks, remove gown, gloves, mask, and cap before leaving the room. *Comments:*	☐	☐	☐	
11. Remove gown using proper technique. Dispose of gown in approved receptacle. *Comments:*	☐	☐	☐	
12. Remove gloves using proper technique. Dispose of gloves in appropriate receptacle. *Comments:*	☐	☐	☐	
13. Remove mask using proper technique and discard. *Comments:*	☐	☐	☐	
14. Removal of cap: Grasp top surface of cap and lift from head. *Comments:*	☐	☐	☐	
15. Wash hands. *Comments:*	☐	☐	☐	
Evaluation				
1. The client remains free of any nosocomial infection. *Comments:*	☐	☐	☐	
2. The health care provider and staff are protected from infection and microorganisms are contained without cross-contamination. *Comments:*	☐	☐	☐	
3. The client interacts on a social level with the nurse, family members, and other visitors. *Comments:*	☐	☐	☐	

Checklist for Procedure 29-3   Taking a Temperature

Name _____   Date _____

School _____

Instructor _____

Course _____

Procedure 29-3 Taking a Temperature	Able to Perform	Able to Perform with Assistance	Unable to Perform	Initials and Date
Assessment				
1. Assess body temperature for changes when exposed to pyrogens (endogenous or exogenous substances that cause fever) or to extreme hot or cold external environments because such environments may indicate the cause of infection. *Comments:*	☐	☐	☐	
2. Assess the client for the most appropriate site to check temperature to obtain an accurate reading. *Comments:*	☐	☐	☐	
3. Confirm that the client has not consumed hot or cold food or beverage nor smoked for 15–30 minutes before the measurement of an oral temperature. *Comments:*	☐	☐	☐	
4. Assess for mouth breathing and tachypnea. *Comments:*	☐	☐	☐	
5. Assess for oral lesions, especially herpetic lesions. *Comments:*	☐	☐	☐	
Planning/Expected Outcomes				
1. An accurate temperature reading will be obtained. *Comments:*	☐	☐	☐	
2. The client will verbalize understanding of the reason for the procedure. *Comments:*	☐	☐	☐	
Implementation				
Preparation				
1. Check client's identification band. Review medical record for baseline data and factors that influence vital signs. *Comments:*	☐	☐	☐	

continued on the following page

continued from the previous page

Procedure 29-3	Able to Perform	Able to Perform with Assistance	Unable to Perform	Initials and Date
2. Explain to the client that vital signs will be assessed. Encourage the client to remain still and refrain from drinking, eating, and smoking and to avoid mouth breathing, if possible. Do not take vital signs within 30 minutes of the client drinking, eating, or smoking as these activities give false readings. *Comments:*	☐	☐	☐	
3. Assess client's toileting needs and proceed as appropriate. *Comments:*	☐	☐	☐	
4. Gather equipment. *Comments:*	☐	☐	☐	
5. Provide for privacy. *Comments:*	☐	☐	☐	
6. Wash hands and apply gloves when appropriate. *Comments:*	☐	☐	☐	
Oral Temperature: Electronic Thermometer				
7. Repeat Actions 1–6. *Comments:*	☐	☐	☐	
8. Place disposable protective sheath over probe. *Comments:*	☐	☐	☐	
9. Grasp top of the probe's stem. Avoid placing pressure on the ejection button. *Comments:*	☐	☐	☐	
10. Place tip of thermometer under the client's tongue and along the gumline to the posterior sublingual pocket lateral to center of the lower jaw. *Comments:*	☐	☐	☐	
11. Instruct client to keep mouth closed around thermometer. *Comments:*	☐	☐	☐	
12. Thermometer will signal (beep) when a constant temperature registers. *Comments:*	☐	☐	☐	

Procedure 29-3	Able to Perform	Able to Perform with Assistance	Unable to Perform	Initials and Date
13. Read measurement on digital display of electronic thermometer. Push ejection button to discard disposable sheath into receptacle and return probe to storage well. *Comments:*	☐	☐	☐	
14. Inform client of temperature reading. *Comments:*	☐	☐	☐	
15. Remove gloves and wash hands. *Comments:*	☐	☐	☐	
16. Record reading according to institution policies. *Comments:*	☐	☐	☐	
17. Return electronic thermometer unit to charging base, checking that it is plugged in. *Comments:*	☐	☐	☐	
18. Wash hands. *Comments:*	☐	☐	☐	
Tympanic Temperature: Infrared Thermometer				
19. Repeat Actions 1–6. *Comments:*	☐	☐	☐	
20. Position client in Sims' or sitting position. *Comments:*	☐	☐	☐	
21. Remove probe from container and attach probe cover to tympanic thermometer unit. *Comments:*	☐	☐	☐	
22. Turn client's head to one side. For an adult, pull pinna upward and back; for a child, pull down and back. Gently insert probe with firm pressure into ear canal. *Comments:*	☐	☐	☐	
23. Remove probe after the reading is displayed on digital unit (usually 2 seconds). *Comments:*	☐	☐	☐	

continued on the following page

continued from the previous page

Procedure 29-3	Able to Perform	Able to Perform with Assistance	Unable to Perform	Initials and Date
24. Discard probe cover into receptacle and replace probe in storage container. *Comments:*	☐	☐	☐	
25. Return tympanic thermometer to storage unit. *Comments:*	☐	☐	☐	
26. Record reading according to institution policy. *Comments:*	☐	☐	☐	
27. Wash hands. *Comments:*	☐	☐	☐	
Using a "Tempa-Dot"				
28. Repeat Actions 1–6. *Comments:*	☐	☐	☐	
29. Position the client in a sitting or lying position. *Comments:*	☐	☐	☐	
30. Prepare Tempa-Dot according to directions (oral or axillary). *Comments:*	☐	☐	☐	
31. Record temperature, indicate the method, and discard the thermometer. *Comments:*	☐	☐	☐	
32. Wash hands. *Comments:*	☐	☐	☐	
Oral Temperature: Plastic Thermometer				
33. Repeat Actions 1–6. *Comments:*	☐	☐	☐	
34. Select correct color tip of thermometer from client's bedside container. *Comments:*	☐	☐	☐	

Procedure 29-3	Able to Perform	Able to Perform with Assistance	Unable to Perform	Initials and Date
35. Remove thermometer from storage container, hold end away from bulb, and rinse under cool water. *Comments:*	☐	☐	☐	
36. Use a tissue to dry thermometer from the bulb's end toward fingertips. *Comments:*	☐	☐	☐	
37. Read thermometer by locating colored solution level. It should read 35.5° C (96° F). *Comments:*	☐	☐	☐	
38. If thermometer is not below normal body temperature reading, grasp thermometer with thumb and forefinger and shake vigorously by snapping the wrist in a downward motion to move colored solution to a level below normal. *Comments:*	☐	☐	☐	
39. Place thermometer in client's mouth under the tongue and along the gumline to the posterior sublingual pocket. Instruct client to hold lips closed. *Comments:*	☐	☐	☐	
40. Leave in place as specified by institution policy, usually 3–5 minutes. *Comments:*	☐	☐	☐	
41. Remove thermometer and wipe with a tissue away from fingers toward the bulb's end. *Comments:*	☐	☐	☐	
42. Read at eye level and rotate slowly until colored solution level is visualized. *Comments:*	☐	☐	☐	
43. Shake thermometer down, cleanse glass thermometer with soapy water, rinse under cold water, and return to storage container. *Comments:*	☐	☐	☐	

continued on the following page

continued from the previous page

Procedure 29-3	Able to Perform	Able to Perform with Assistance	Unable to Perform	Initials and Date
44. Remove and dispose of gloves in receptacle. Wash hands. *Comments:*	☐	☐	☐	
45. Record reading according to institution policy. *Comments:*	☐	☐	☐	
46. Wash hands. *Comments:*	☐	☐	☐	
Rectal Temperature 47. Repeat Actions 1–6. *Comments:*	☐	☐	☐	
48. Place client in the Sims' position with upper knee flexed. Adjust sheet to expose only anal area. *Comments:*	☐	☐	☐	
49. Place tissues in easy reach. Apply gloves. *Comments:*	☐	☐	☐	
50. Prepare the thermometer. *Comments:*	☐	☐	☐	
51. Lubricate sheath or probe covering tip of rectal thermometer (a rectal thermometer usually has a red tip or cap). *Comments:*	☐	☐	☐	
52. With dominant hand, grasp thermometer. With other hand, separate buttocks to expose anus. *Comments:*	☐	☐	☐	
53. Instruct client to take a deep breath. Insert thermometer or probe gently into anus: infant, 1.2 cm (0.5 inches); adult, 3.5 cm (1.5 inches). If resistance is felt, do not force insertion. *Comments:*	☐	☐	☐	
54. Hold plastic thermometer in place for 3–5 minutes. If taking the rectal temperature with an electronic probe, remove it after the reading is displayed on digital unit (usually 2 seconds). *Comments:*	☐	☐	☐	

Procedure 29-3	Able to Perform	Able to Perform with Assistance	Unable to Perform	Initials and Date
55. Wipe off secretions on the plastic thermometer with a tissue. Dispose of tissue in a receptacle. *Comments:*	☐	☐	☐	
56. Read measurement and inform client of temperature reading. *Comments:*	☐	☐	☐	
57. While holding glass thermometer in one hand, use other hand to wipe anal area with tissue to remove lubricant or feces. Dispose of soiled tissue. Cover client. *Comments:*	☐	☐	☐	
58. Wash thermometer. *Comments:*	☐	☐	☐	
59. Remove and dispose of gloves in receptacle. Wash hands. *Comments:*	☐	☐	☐	
60. Record reading according to institution policy. *Comments:*	☐	☐	☐	
Axillary Temperature				
61. Repeat Actions 1–6. *Comments:*	☐	☐	☐	
62. Remove client's arm and shoulder from sleeve of gown. Avoid exposing chest. *Comments:*	☐	☐	☐	
63. Make sure axillary skin is dry; if necessary, pat dry. *Comments:*	☐	☐	☐	
64. Prepare thermometer. *Comments:*	☐	☐	☐	
65. Place thermometer or probe into center of axilla. Fold the client's upper arm straight down, and place arm across client's chest. On a thin client, make sure flesh rather than hollow armpit surrounds the thermometer or probe. *Comments:*	☐	☐	☐	

continued on the following page

continued from the previous page

Procedure 29-3	Able to Perform	Able to Perform with Assistance	Unable to Perform	Initials and Date
66. Leave glass thermometer in place as specified by institution policy (usually 6–8 minutes). Leave an electronic thermometer in place until signal is heard. *Comments:*	☐	☐	☐	
67. Remove and read thermometer. *Comments:*	☐	☐	☐	
68. Inform client of temperature reading. *Comments:*	☐	☐	☐	
69. If using a thermometer, shake down the solution. Wash glass thermometer with soapy water, rinse under cold water, and return to storage container. If using an electric thermometer, push ejection button to discard disposable sheath into receptacle and return probe to storage well. *Comments:*	☐	☐	☐	
70. Assist the client with replacing the gown. *Comments:*	☐	☐	☐	
71. Record reading according to institution policy. *Comments:*	☐	☐	☐	
72. Wash hands. *Comments:*	☐	☐	☐	
Disposable (Chemical Strip) Thermometer				
73. Repeat Actions 1–6. *Comments:*	☐	☐	☐	
74. Apply tape to appropriate skin area, usually forehead. *Comments:*	☐	☐	☐	
75. Observe tape for color changes. *Comments:*	☐	☐	☐	
76. Record reading and indicate method. *Comments:*	☐	☐	☐	

Procedure 29-3	Able to Perform	Able to Perform with Assistance	Unable to Perform	Initials and Date
77. Wash hands. *Comments:*	☐	☐	☐	
Noninvasive Temporal Artery Scan Thermometer (Temporal Scanner)				
78. Repeat Actions 1–6. *Comments:*	☐	☐	☐	
79. Locate the client's exposed temporal artery. *Comments:*	☐	☐	☐	
80. Place the thermometer sensor head in the center of the forehead halfway between the eyebrows and the hairline. *Comments:*	☐	☐	☐	
81. Slide the thermometer straight across the forehead stopping at the hairline. *Comments:*	☐	☐	☐	
82. Record reading and indicate method. *Comments:*	☐	☐	☐	
83. Wash hands. *Comments:*	☐	☐	☐	
Evaluation				
1. Establish client's baseline temperature. *Comments:*	☐	☐	☐	
2. Compare temperature with the client's baseline temperature. *Comments:*	☐	☐	☐	
3. Evaluate the client's condition for trauma caused by the instrument. *Comments:*	☐	☐	☐	

Checklist for Procedure 29-4   Taking a Pulse

Name _____ Date _____

School _____

Instructor _____

Course _____

Procedure 29-4 Taking a Pulse	Able to Perform	Able to Perform with Assistance	Unable to Perform	Initials and Date
Assessment				
1. Assess client for need to monitor pulse. *Comments:*	☐	☐	☐	
2. Assess the pulse for rate, amplitude (volume, strength), and regularity to determine the heart's pumping action and the adequacy of peripheral artery blood flow. *Comments:*	☐	☐	☐	
3. Assess for signs and symptoms of cardiovascular alterations, such as dyspnea, chest pain, orthopnea, syncope, palpitations, edema of extremities, cyanosis, or fatigue, because these signs may indicate deficient cardiac or vascular function. *Comments:*	☐	☐	☐	
4. Assess client for factors that may affect the character of the pulse, such as age, medications, exercise, change in position, or fever. *Comments:*	☐	☐	☐	
5. Assess for the appropriate site for measuring pulse so the pulse will be accurate. *Comments:*	☐	☐	☐	
6. Assess baseline heart rate and rhythm in the client's chart to compare it with the current measurement. *Comments:*	☐	☐	☐	
7. Assess circulatory status by using appropriate site because pulses may be affected by surgery, medical condition, arterial blood draws, or poor circulation. *Comments:*	☐	☐	☐	

continued on the following page

continued from the previous page

Procedure 29-4	Able to Perform	Able to Perform with Assistance	Unable to Perform	Initials and Date
Planning/Expected Outcomes				
1. Pulse rate, quality, rhythm, and volume will be within normal range for the client's age group. *Comments:*	☐	☐	☐	
2. The client will be comfortable with the procedure and demonstrate an understanding regarding its importance. *Comments:*	☐	☐	☐	
Implementation				
Taking a Radial (Wrist) Pulse				
1. Check client's identification band. Explain procedure before beginning. Wash hands. *Comments:*	☐	☐	☐	
2. Inform client of the site(s) at which you will measure pulse. *Comments:*	☐	☐	☐	
3. Flex client's elbow and place lower part of arm across chest. *Comments:*	☐	☐	☐	
4. Support client's wrist by grasping outer aspect with thumb. *Comments:*	☐	☐	☐	
5. Place your index and middle fingers on inner aspect of client's wrist over the radial artery and apply light but firm pressure until pulse is palpated. *Comments:*	☐	☐	☐	
6. Identify pulse rhythm or regularity. *Comments:*	☐	☐	☐	
7. Determine pulse volume or amplitude. *Comments:*	☐	☐	☐	
8. Count pulse rate by using second hand on a watch. *Comments:*	☐	☐	☐	
Taking an Apical Pulse				
9. Wash hands. *Comments:*	☐	☐	☐	

Procedure 29-4	Able to Perform	Able to Perform with Assistance	Unable to Perform	Initials and Date
10. Raise client's gown to expose sternum and left side of chest. *Comments:*	☐	☐	☐	
11. Cleanse earpiece and diaphragm of stethoscope with an alcohol swab. *Comments:*	☐	☐	☐	
12. Put stethoscope around your neck. *Comments:*	☐	☐	☐	
13. Locate apex of heart. *Comments:*	☐	☐	☐	
14. Inform client you are going to listen to his or her heart. Instruct client to remain silent. *Comments:*	☐	☐	☐	
15. With dominant hand, put earpiece of the stethoscope in your ears and grasp diaphragm of the stethoscope in palm of your hand for 5–10 seconds. *Comments:*	☐	☐	☐	
16. Place diaphragm of stethoscope over the apical impulse and auscultate for sounds S1 and S2 to hear lub-dub sound. *Comments:*	☐	☐	☐	
17. Note regularity of rhythm. *Comments:*	☐	☐	☐	
18. Start to count while looking at second hand or digital display of watch. *Comments:*	☐	☐	☐	
19. Share your findings with client. *Comments:*	☐	☐	☐	
20. Record by site the rate, rhythm, and, if applicable, number of irregular beats. *Comments:*	☐	☐	☐	

continued on the following page

continued from the previous page

Procedure 29-4	Able to Perform	Able to Perform with Assistance	Unable to Perform	Initials and Date
21. Wash hands. *Comments:*	☐	☐	☐	
Evaluation				
1. Compare client's pulse with baseline rate, amplitude (volume, strength), and rhythm (regularity) to detect any changes. *Comments:*	☐	☐	☐	
2. If pulse is irregular or abnormal, ask another nurse to check the pulse and then report to health care provider. *Comments:*	☐	☐	☐	
3. Evaluate pulse site as required by client's condition and compare bilateral pulses. *Comments:*	☐	☐	☐	

Checklist for Procedure 29-5   Counting Respirations

Name _____ Date _____

School _____

Instructor _____

Course _____

Procedure 29-5 Counting Respirations	Able to Perform	Able to Perform with Assistance	Unable to Perform	Initials and Date
Assessment				
1. Assess the the movement client's chest wall to see if it is equal bilaterally, if the movement is labored, or if the client is using accessory muscles to breathe. *Comments:*	☐	☐	☐	
2. Assess the rate of respirations to identify slow, rapid, or irregular respirations or even periods of apnea. *Comments:*	☐	☐	☐	
3. Assess the depth of the client's breaths to monitor shallow, deep, or uneven respirations. Think if there might be something influencing the client's respirations. Is the client in pain, frightened, talking, or smoking? *Comments:*	☐	☐	☐	
4. Assess for risk factors such as fever, pain, anxiety, diseases, or trauma to the chest wall that may alter the respirations because certain conditions may cause increased risk of alterations in respirations. *Comments:*	☐	☐	☐	
5. Assess for factors that normally influence respirations, such as age, exercise, anxiety, pain, smoking, medications, or postural changes, so that an accurate assessment can be made. *Comments:*	☐	☐	☐	
Planning/Expected Outcomes				
1. An accurate evaluation of a client's respiratory rate and character is obtained. *Comments:*	☐	☐	☐	
2. The respiratory rate and character is normal. *Comments:*	☐	☐	☐	

continued on the following page

continued from the previous page

Procedure 29-5	Able to Perform	Able to Perform with Assistance	Unable to Perform	Initials and Date
Implementation				
1. Check client's identification band. Explain procedure before beginning. Wash hands. *Comments:*	☐	☐	☐	
2. Be sure chest movement is visible. Client may need to remove heavy clothing. *Comments:*	☐	☐	☐	
3. Observe one complete respiratory cycle. *Comments:*	☐	☐	☐	
4. Start counting with first inspiration while looking at the second hand of watch. (For infants and children: count full minute; Adults: count for 30 seconds and multiply by 2. If an irregular rate/rhythm is present, count for 1 full minute.) *Comments:*	☐	☐	☐	
5. Observe character of respirations (depth and rhythm). *Comments:*	☐	☐	☐	
6. Observe skin color and level of consciousness. *Comments:*	☐	☐	☐	
7. Replace client's gown if needed. *Comments:*	☐	☐	☐	
8. Record rate and character of respirations. *Comments:*	☐	☐	☐	
9. Wash hands. *Comments:*	☐	☐	☐	
Evaluation				
1. Evaluate client's respirations as a baseline value. *Comments:*	☐	☐	☐	
2. Compare respirations with baseline to detect any alterations. *Comments:*	☐	☐	☐	

Checklist for Procedure 29-6   Taking Blood Pressure

Name _____ Date _____

School _____

Instructor _____

Course _____

Procedure 29-6 Taking Blood Pressure	Able to Perform	Able to Perform with Assistance	Unable to Perform	Initials and Date
Assessment				
1. Assess the condition of the potential blood pressure (BP) site so that a site with an injury or surgery proximal to the site can be avoided. *Comments:*	☐	☐	☐	
2. Assess the artery for any compromise to it so that compressing the artery briefly will not cause decrease in circulation. *Comments:*	☐	☐	☐	
3. Assess the distal pulse to check if it is intact and palpable. *Comments:*	☐	☐	☐	
4. Assess the circumference of the extremity for the right size cuff so an accurate reading can be obtained. *Comments:*	☐	☐	☐	
5. Assess for factors that affect blood pressure, such as age, fear, anxiety, medications, smoking, eating or exercising within 30 minutes prior to BP assessment, and postural changes so an accurate reading can be obtained. *Comments:*	☐	☐	☐	
6. Determine client's baseline blood pressure by reading the medical record so a comparison can be made with each BP reading. *Comments:*	☐	☐	☐	
Planning/Expected Outcomes				
1. An accurate estimate of the arterial pressure at diastole and systole is obtained. *Comments:*	☐	☐	☐	
2. Blood pressure is within the expected range for the client. *Comments:*	☐	☐	☐	

continued on the following page

continued from the previous page

Procedure 29-6	**Able to Perform**	**Able to Perform with Assistance**	**Unable to Perform**	**Initials and Date**
3. Client understands why the blood pressure is taken and what it means. *Comments:*	☐	☐	☐	

Implementation

Auscultation Method Using Brachial Artery

	Able to Perform	**Able to Perform with Assistance**	**Unable to Perform**	**Initials and Date**
1. Check client's identification band. Explain procedure before beginning. Wash hands. *Comments:*	☐	☐	☐	
2. Determine which extremity is most appropriate for reading. Do not take a pressure reading on an injured or painful extremity or one in which an intravenous line is running. *Comments:*	☐	☐	☐	
3. Select a cuff size appropriate for the client. Estimate by inspections, or measure with a tape, the circumference of the bare upper arm at the midpoint between the shoulder (acromion) and the elbow (olecranon process). *Comments:*	☐	☐	☐	
4. Have the client's bared arm resting on a support so the midpoint of the upper arm is at the level of the heart. Extend the elbow with the palm turned upward. *Comments:*	☐	☐	☐	
5. Make sure bladder cuff is fully deflated and the pump valve moves freely. Place the manometer so that the center of the aneroid dial is at eye level and easily visible to the observer. *Comments:*	☐	☐	☐	
6. Palpate brachial artery, in the antecubital space, and place the cuff so that the midline of the bladder is over the arterial pulsation. Next, wrap and secure the cuff snugly around the client's bare upper arm. The lower edge of the cuff should be 1 inch (2 cm) above the antecubital fossa (bend of the elbow). *Comments:*	☐	☐	☐	

Procedure 29-6	Able to Perform	Able to Perform with Assistance	Unable to Perform	Initials and Date
7. Inflate cuff rapidly to 70 mm Hg and increase by 10-mm increments while palpating the radial pulse. Note the level of pressure at which the pulse disappears and subsequently reappears during deflation. Let all of the air out of the cuff in preparation for reinflating the cuff to take the BP reading. Let the arm rest 1 minute before reinflating the cuff. This is called the two-step method of obtaining a BP by obtaining a baseline prior to obtaining the BP reading. *Comments:*	☐	☐	☐	
8. Insert the earpieces of the stethoscope into the ear canals with a forward tilt to fit snugly. *Comments:*	☐	☐	☐	
9. Relocate the brachial artery with your nondominate hand and place the bell of the stethoscope over the brachial artery pulsation. *Comments:*	☐	☐	☐	
10. With your dominant hand, turn the valve clockwise to close. Compress the pump to inflate the cuff rapidly and steadily until the manometer registers 20 to 30 mm Hg above the level previously determined by the palpation. *Comments:*	☐	☐	☐	
11. Partially unscrew (open) the valve counterclockwise to deflate the bladder at 2 mm/sec while listening for the appearance of the five phases of the Korotkoff sounds. *Comments:*	☐	☐	☐	
12. After the last Korotkoff sound is heard, deflate the cuff slowly for at least another 10 mm Hg to ensure that no other sounds are audible; then, deflate rapidly and completely. *Comments:*	☐	☐	☐	
13. Allow the client to rest for at least 30 seconds and remove cuff. *Comments:*	☐	☐	☐	
14. Inform the client of the reading. *Comments:*	☐	☐	☐	

continued on the following page

continued from the previous page

Procedure 29-6	Able to Perform	Able to Perform with Assistance	Unable to Perform	Initials and Date
15. The systolic (Phase 5) pressure should be immediately recorded, rounded off (upward) to the nearest 2 mm Hg. In children and when sounds are heard to the level of 0 mm Hg, the Phase 4 pressure should also be recorded. *Comments:*	☐	☐	☐	
16. If appropriate, lower bed and place call light in easy reach. *Comments:*	☐	☐	☐	
17. Put all equipment in proper place. *Comments:*	☐	☐	☐	
18. Wash hands. *Comments:*	☐	☐	☐	
Evaluation				
1. Evaluate the BP reading for accuracy by comparing with the medical record. *Comments:*	☐	☐	☐	
2. Evaluate the client's BP for being within the normal range. *Comments:*	☐	☐	☐	
3. Identify variations in the client's BP of more than 5–10 mm Hg from one arm to the other. *Comments:*	☐	☐	☐	
4. Evaluate if the client's BP changes significantly when he or she stands up. *Comments:*	☐	☐	☐	
5. Report abnormal measurements to charge nurse or health care provider. *Comments:*	☐	☐	☐	

Checklist for Procedure 29-7   Performing Pulse Oximetry

Name _____ Date _____

School _____

Instructor _____

Course _____

Procedure 29-7 Performing Pulse Oximetry	Able to Perform	Able to Perform with Assistance	Unable to Perform	Initials and Date
Assessment				
1. Assess the client's hemoglobin level. Because pulse oximetry measures the percent of SaO_2, the results of the oxygenation status are affected. The results appear normal if the hemoglobin level is low because all hemoglobin available to carry O_2 is completely saturated; therefore, it is important to know the hemoglobin level *Comments:*	☐	☐	☐	
2. Assess the client's color. If the client has vasoconstriction of the extremities, an inaccurate recording may be obtained. *Comments:*	☐	☐	☐	
3. Assess the client's mental status as this assists in general evaluation of oxygen delivery to the brain and indicates a high level of CO_2. *Comments:*	☐	☐	☐	
4. Assess the client's pulse rate. The pulse oximeter measures pulse rate. Manually assessing the pulse is a cross-reference to indicate functioning of the oximeter. *Comments:*	☐	☐	☐	
5. Assess the area where the sensors are placed to determine whether it is an area with adequate circulation (no scars or thickened nails). *Comments:*	☐	☐	☐	
6. Remove any nail polish or acrylic nails, which interfere with sensor measurements. *Comments:*	☐	☐	☐	

continued on the following page

continued from the previous page

Procedure 29-7	Able to Perform	Able to Perform with Assistance	Unable to Perform	Initials and Date
Planning/Expected Outcomes				
1. The SaO$_2$ will be in a normal range for the client (95%–100% in the absence of chronic respiratory disease). *Comments:*	☐	☐	☐	
2. The client will be alert and oriented. *Comments:*	☐	☐	☐	
3. The client's color will remain normal. *Comments:*	☐	☐	☐	
4. The client will tolerate the placement of sensors. *Comments:*	☐	☐	☐	
5. There will not be any skin irritation or pressure from sensors. *Comments:*	☐	☐	☐	
Implementation				
1. Check client's identification band. Explain procedure before beginning. Wash hands. *Comments:*	☐	☐	☐	
2. Select an appropriate sensor. Sensors are commonly used for the fingertips. *Comments:*	☐	☐	☐	
3. Select an appropriate site for the sensor. Fingers are most commonly used; however, toes, earlobes, nose, forehead, hands, and feet are also used. Assess for capillary refill and proximal pulse. If the client has poor circulation, use an earlobe, forehead, or nasal sensor instead. In children, sensors are used on the hand, foot, or trunk. If elderly clients have thickened nails, pick another site. *Comments:*	☐	☐	☐	
4. Clean the site with an alcohol wipe. Remove artificial nails or nail polish if present or select another site. Clean any tape adhesive. Use soap and water if necessary to clean the site. *Comments:*	☐	☐	☐	

Procedure 29-7	Able to Perform	Able to Perform with Assistance	Unable to Perform	Initials and Date
5. Apply the sensor. Make sure the photon detectors are aligned on opposite sides of the selected site. *Comments:*	☐	☐	☐	
6. Connect the sensor to the oximeter with a sensor cable. Turn on the machine. Initially a tone is heard, followed by an arterial wave-form fluctuation with each arterial pulse. In most oximeters, if the battery is low, a low-battery light illuminates when 15 minutes of battery life are remaining. Plug in oximeters even when not in use. *Comments:*	☐	☐	☐	
7. Adjust the alarm limits for high and low O_2 saturation levels according to the manufacturer's directions. Pulse rate limits are usually set. Adjust volume. *Comments:*	☐	☐	☐	
8. If taking a reading, note the results. If the oximeter is being used for constant monitoring, move the site of spring sensors every 2 hours and adhesive sensors every 4 hours. *Comments:*	☐	☐	☐	
9. Cover the sensor with a sheet or towel to protect it from exposure to bright light. *Comments:*	☐	☐	☐	
10. If abnormal results are obtained, first assess the client. Are client's hands cold? Is the sensor correctly placed on the client's finger? Is the oximetry device broken? Obtain the pulse oximetry with another device. If the results are still abnormal, notify the health care provider of abnormal results. *Comments:*	☐	☐	☐	
11. Wash hands. *Comments:*	☐	☐	☐	

Evaluation

	Able to Perform	Able to Perform with Assistance	Unable to Perform	Initials and Date
1. The SaO_2 is in the normal range for the client (95%–100% in the absence of chronic respiratory disease). *Comments:*	☐	☐	☐	

continued on the following page

continued from the previous page

Procedure 29-7	Able to Perform	Able to Perform with Assistance	Unable to Perform	Initials and Date
2. The client is alert and oriented. *Comments:*	☐	☐	☐	
3. The client's color is normal. *Comments:*	☐	☐	☐	
4. The client tolerates the placement of sensors. *Comments:*	☐	☐	☐	
5. There is no skin irritation or pressure from sensors. *Comments:*	☐	☐	☐	

Checklist for Procedure 29-8   Weighing a Client, Mobile and Immobile

Name _____ Date _____

School _____

Instructor _____

Course _____

Procedure 29-8 Weighing a Client, Mobile and Immobile	Able to Perform	Able to Perform with Assistance	Unable to Perform	Initials and Date
Assessment				
1. Assess the client's ability to stand independently and safely on a scale. Consider factors requiring the use of a sling: The client is somnolent or comatose, paralyzed, too weak to stand, or unsteady when standing. *Comments:*	☐	☐	☐	
2. Determine if clothing is similar to that worn during previous weight measurement to help determine accuracy of the new weight. *Comments:*	☐	☐	☐	
Planning/Expected Outcomes				
1. Health care provider obtains accurate weight. *Comments:*	☐	☐	☐	
2. Client incurs no injuries. *Comments:*	☐	☐	☐	
3. Client maintains privacy. *Comments:*	☐	☐	☐	
Implementation				
Standing Scale 1. Check client's identification band. Explain procedure before beginning. Wash hands. *Comments:*	☐	☐	☐	
2. Place the scale near the client. *Comments:*	☐	☐	☐	
3. Turn on the electronic scale and calibrate scale to zero. *Comments :*	☐	☐	☐	

continued on the following page

continued from the previous page

Procedure 29-8	Able to Perform	Able to Perform with Assistance	Unable to Perform	Initials and Date
4. Ask client to remove shoes if necessary, step up on the scale and stand still. *Electronic scale*: Read weight after digital numbers have stopped fluctuating. *Balance scale*: Slide the larger weight into the notch most closely approximating the client's weight. Slide the smaller weight into the notch so the balance rests in the middle. Add the two numbers for the client's weight. *Comments:*	☐	☐	☐	
5. Ask client to step down. Assist the client back to the bed or chair, if necessary. *Comments:*	☐	☐	☐	
6. Wipe the scale with appropriate disinfectant. *Comments:*	☐	☐	☐	
7. Wash hands. *Comments:*	☐	☐	☐	
Sling Scale				
8. Wash hands and put on gloves if needed. *Comments:*	☐	☐	☐	
9. Place plastic covering on sling if available (can usually be ordered in bulk from the manufacturer). *Comments:*	☐	☐	☐	
10. Remove pillows. Turn the client to one side and place half of sling on bed next to the client, with remaining half rolled up against the client's back. *Comments:*	☐	☐	☐	
11. Turn the client to other side, and unroll the rest of the sling so it lays flat beneath the client. *Comments:*	☐	☐	☐	
12. Roll the scale over the bed so the legs of the scale are underneath the bed. Open and lock the legs of the scale. *Comments:*	☐	☐	☐	
13. Turn on scale and calibrate to zero. *Comments:*	☐	☐	☐	

Procedure 29-8	Able to Perform	Able to Perform with Assistance	Unable to Perform	Initials and Date
14. Lower arms of the scale and slip hooks through holes in sling. Comments:	☐	☐	☐	
15. Pump scale until sling rests completely off the bed. Comments:	☐	☐	☐	
16. Remind the client to remain still. Read weight after digital numbers have stopped fluctuating. Comments:	☐	☐	☐	
17. Lower client back to bed and remove arms of the scale from sling. Comments:	☐	☐	☐	
18. Unlock scale legs, return to their original position, and remove scale from bed. Comments:	☐	☐	☐	
19. Turn the client on his or her side to side, roll up sling, and then turn client to the other side. Comments:	☐	☐	☐	
20. Realign the client with pillows and covers. Comments:	☐	☐	☐	
21. Remove plastic covering from the sling and discard as per hospital policy. Comments:	☐	☐	☐	
22. Remove gloves and wash hands. Comments:	☐	☐	☐	
Bed Scale or Under Bed Pod Scale				
23. Place the same amount of bedding on the bed and clothing on the client. Comments:	☐	☐	☐	
24. Turn on electronic weight monitor and weigh client. Comments:	☐	☐	☐	

continued on the following page

continued from the previous page

Procedure 29-8	**Able to Perform**	**Able to Perform with Assistance**	**Unable to Perform**	**Initials and Date**
Evaluation				
1. Compare weight obtained to previously recorded weight. Repeat weight if large discrepancy is noted. *Comments:*	☐	☐	☐	
2. If large discrepancy still remains, notify appropriate health care team members. *Comments:*	☐	☐	☐	

Checklist for Procedure 29-9   Proper Body Mechanics

Name _____   Date _____

School _____

Instructor _____

Course _____

Procedure 29-9 **Proper Body Mechanics**	Able to Perform	Able to Perform with Assistance	Unable to Perform	Initials and Date
Assessment				
1. Assess the need and degree to which the client requires assistance to achieve physical movement. Identifies client's ability to attain maximum level of self-help before initiating intervention. *Comments:*	☐	☐	☐	
2. Identify the type of physical movement required to ensure the use of proper body mechanics such as pushing, pulling, or lifting. *Comments:*	☐	☐	☐	
3. Identify the potential need for assistive equipment to accomplish the goal of safe lifting and to minimize the risk of client or nurse injury. *Comments:*	☐	☐	☐	
4. Identify any unusual risks to safe lifting, such as an extra-heavy client or a home care setting. Plan modifications if needed to ensure good body mechanics and reduce the risk of injury. *Comments:*	☐	☐	☐	
5. Assess the situation for obstacles, heavy clients, poor handholds, and equipment or objects in the way. Reduce or remove safety hazards prior to lifting the client or object. *Comments:*	☐	☐	☐	
6. Assess the situation for slippery surfaces, including wet floors; slippery shoes on client, helper, or nurse; and towels, linen, or paper on the floor. Resolve the slippery surface before lifting the client or object. *Comments:*	☐	☐	☐	

continued on the following page

continued from the previous page

Procedure 29-9	Able to Perform	Able to Perform with Assistance	Unable to Perform	Initials and Date
7. Assess the situation for hidden risks, including client confusion, combativeness, orthostatic hypotension, drug effects, pain, or fear. *Comments:*	☐	☐	☐	
8. Assess the client's vital signs, pain status, and need for pain medications before ambulating. Assess incisional areas and/or areas of injury. *Comments:*	☐	☐	☐	
9. Check equipment to ensure that it is in working order to facilitate a safe and uninterrupted transfer. Especially check locks on wheelchair. *Comments:*	☐	☐	☐	
10. Identify all equipment and tubes connected to the client and take appropriate preventive measures. Frequently, clients who require lifting or transfer have intravenous tubing, other tubing, and/or orthopedic equipment. *Comments:*	☐	☐	☐	
11. Assess the client's understanding of the steps required to achieve the goal of a safe transfer and the ability to assist. Explanation of the steps in a clear, concise fashion will decrease anxiety, secure cooperation, and ease physical requirements for both the client and the nurse or caregiver. *Comments:*	☐	☐	☐	
Planning/Expected Outcomes				
1. Client is safely lifted/transferred by staff utilizing appropriate equipment and correct body mechanics. *Comments:*	☐	☐	☐	
2. Accidents during lifting of client are avoided by using proper body alignment and mechanics. *Comments:*	☐	☐	☐	
3. Heavy lifting is facilitated by mechanical devices and a team effort. *Comments:*	☐	☐	☐	

Procedure 29-9	Able to Perform	Able to Perform with Assistance	Unable to Perform	Initials and Date
4. Client and family are taught safe lifting/transfer techniques to facilitate this process in home and extended-care environments. *Comments:*	☐	☐	☐	
5. The nurse practices safe lifting and proper body mechanics when performing nursing care that requires bending or lifting. *Comments:*	☐	☐	☐	
6. Staff and clients are not injured using correct body mechanics and appropriate equipment. *Comments:*	☐	☐	☐	
Implementation				
1. Check the client's identification band. Explain procedure before beginning. Wash hands. *Comments:*	☐	☐	☐	
2. Assess the client situation as stated in Assessment section for this procedure. *Comments:*	☐	☐	☐	
3. Maintain low center of gravity by bending at the hips and knees, not at the waist. Squat down rather than bend over to lift and lower. *Comments:*	☐	☐	☐	
4. Establish a wide support base with feet spread apart. *Comments:*	☐	☐	☐	
5. Use feet to move, not a twisting or bending motion from the waist. *Comments:*	☐	☐	☐	
6. When pushing or pulling, stand near the object and stagger one foot partially ahead of the other. *Comments:*	☐	☐	☐	
7. When pushing a client or an object, lean into the client or object and apply continuous light pressure. When pulling a client or an object, lean away and grasp with light pressure. Never jerk or twist your body to force a weight to move. *Comments:*	☐	☐	☐	

continued on the following page

continued from the previous page

Procedure 29-9	Able to Perform	Able to Perform with Assistance	Unable to Perform	Initials and Date
8. When stooping to move an object, maintain a wide base of support with feet, flex knees to lower, and maintain straight upper body. *Comments:*	☐	☐	☐	
9. When lifting or carrying an object, squat down in front of the object, take a firm hold, and assume a standing position by using the leg muscles and keeping the back straight. *Comments:*	☐	☐	☐	
10. When raising up from a squatting position, arch your back slightly. Keep the buttocks and abdomen tucked in and raise up with your head first. *Comments:*	☐	☐	☐	
11. When lifting or carrying heavy objects, keep the weight as close to your center of gravity as possible. *Comments:*	☐	☐	☐	
12. When reaching for a client or an object, keep the back straight. If the client or object is heavy, do not try to lift the client or object without repositioning yourself closer to the weight. *Comments:*	☐	☐	☐	
13. Use safety aids and equipment. Use gait belts, lifts, drawsheets, and other transfer assistance devices. Encourage clients to use handrails and grab bars. Wheelchair, cart, and stretcher wheels are locked when they are not actually being moved. *Comments:*	☐	☐	☐	
Evaluation				
1. The client or object is lifted and moved without sustaining injury or damage. *Comments:*	☐	☐	☐	
2. The nurse who is lifting and moving clients or objects is not injured. *Comments:*	☐	☐	☐	

Checklist for Procedure 29-10   Performing Passive Range-of-Motion (ROM) Exercises

Name _____ Date _____

School _____

Instructor _____

Course _____

Procedure 29-10 Performing Passive Range-of-Motion (ROM) Exercises	Able to Perform	Able to Perform with Assistance	Unable to Perform	Initials and Date
Assessment				
1. Be aware of the client's medical diagnosis. Understand the expected functional limits of a client with this diagnosis. Comments:	☐	☐	☐	
2. Familiarize yourself with the client's current range of motion. Note any joint pain, stiffness, or inflammation that might limit the client's motion. Comments:	☐	☐	☐	
3. Assess client consciousness and cognitive function. Encourage client to participate in ROM as actively as possible. Comments:	☐	☐	☐	
Planning/Expected Outcomes				
1. Client will maintain or improve current functional mobility in all involved joints and extremities. Comments:	☐	☐	☐	
2. Client will regain or improve strength and/or voluntary movement in involved joints and extremities. Comments:	☐	☐	☐	
3. Client will avoid complications of immobility, including pressure ulcers, contractures, decreased peristalsis, constipation, fecal impactions, orthostatic hypotension, pulmonary embolism, and thrombophlebitis. Comments:	☐	☐	☐	
Implementation				
1. Wash hands, check client's identification band, explain procedure, and wear gloves if contact with body fluids is possible. Comments:	☐	☐	☐	

continued on the following page

continued from the previous page

Procedure 29-10	Able to Perform	Able to Perform with Assistance	Unable to Perform	Initials and Date
2. Provide for privacy, including exposing only the extremity to be exercised. *Comments:*	☐	☐	☐	
3. Adjust bed to comfortable height for performing ROM. *Comments:*	☐	☐	☐	
4. Lower bed rail only on the side you are working. *Comments:*	☐	☐	☐	
5. Describe the passive ROM exercises you are performing or verbally cue client to perform ROM exercises with your assistance. *Comments:*	☐	☐	☐	
6. Start at the client's head and perform ROM exercises down each side of the body. *Comments:*	☐	☐	☐	
7. Repeat each ROM exercise three to five times as the client tolerates, with five times as maximum. Perform each motion in a slow, firm manner. Encourage full joint movement but do not go beyond the point of pain, resistance, or fatigue. *Comments:*	☐	☐	☐	
8. Perform the following movements: a. *Temporomandibular Joint (TMJ)* *(Synovial Joint)* • Open mouth. • Close mouth. • Protrusion: Push out lower jaw. • Retrusion: Tuck in lower jaw. • Lateral motion: Slide jaw from side to side. *Comments:*	☐	☐	☐	
b. *Cervical Spine (Pivot Joint)* • Flexion: Rest chin on chest. • Extension: Return head to midline. • Hyperextension: Tilt head back. • Lateral flexion: Move head to touch ear to shoulder. • Rotation: Turn head to look to side. *Comments:*	☐	☐	☐	

Procedure 29-10	Able to Perform	Able to Perform with Assistance	Unable to Perform	Initials and Date
c. *Shoulder (Ball-and-Socket Joint)* • Flexion: Raise straight arm forward to a position above head. • Extension: Return straight arm forward and down to side of body. • Hyperextension: Move straight arm behind body. • Abduction: Move straight arm downward laterally from side to a position above the head, palm facing away from head. • Adduction: Move straight arm downward laterally across front of body as far as possible. • Circumduction: Move straight arm in a full circle. • External rotation: Bent arm lateral, parallel to floor, palm down, rotate shoulder so fingers point up. • Internal rotation: Bent arm lateral, parallel to floor, rotate shoulder so fingers point down. *Comments:*	☐	☐	☐	
d. *Elbow (Hinge Joint)* • Flexion: Bend elbow, move lower arm toward shoulder, palm facing shoulder. • Extension: Straighten lower arm forward and downward. • Rotation for supination: Elbow bent, turn hand and forearm so palm is facing upward. • Rotation for pronation: Elbow bent, turn hand and forearm so palm is facing downward. *Comments:*	☐	☐	☐	
e. *Wrist (Condyloid Joint)* • Flexion: Bend wrist so fingers move toward inner aspect of forearm. • Extension: Straighten hand to same plane arm. • Hyperextension: Bend wrist so fingers move back as far as possible. • Radial flexion–abduction: Bend wrist laterally toward thumb. • Ulnar flexion–adduction: Bend wrist laterally away from thumb. *Comments:*	☐	☐	☐	

continued on the following page

continued from the previous page

Procedure 29-10	**Able to Perform**	**Able to Perform with Assistance**	**Unable to Perform**	**Initials and Date**
f. *Hand and Fingers (Condyloid and Hinge Joints)* • Flexion: Make a fist. • Extension: Straighten fingers. • Hyperextension: Bend fingers back as far as possible. • Abduction: Spread fingers apart. • Adduction: Bring fingers together. *Comments:*	☐	☐	☐	
g. *Thumb (Saddle Joint)* • Flexion: Move thumb across palmer surface of hand. • Extension: Move thumb away from hand. • Abduction: Move thumb laterally. • Adduction: Move thumb back to hand. • Opposition: Touch thumb to tip of each finger of same hand. *Comments:*	☐	☐	☐	
h. *Hip (Ball-and-Socket Joint)* • Flexion: Move straight leg forward and upward. • Extension: Move leg back beside the other leg. • Hyperextension: Move leg behind body. • Abduction: Move leg laterally from midline. • Adduction: Move leg back past midline. • Circumduction: Move leg backward in a circle. • Internal rotation: Turn foot and leg inward, pointing toes toward other leg. • External rotation: Turn foot and leg outward, pointing toes away from other leg. *Comments:*	☐	☐	☐	
i. *Knee (Hinge Joint)* • Flexion: Bend knee to bring heel back toward thigh. • Extension: Straighten leg, place foot beside other foot. *Comments:*	☐	☐	☐	
j. *Ankle (Hinge Joint)* • Plantar flexion: Point toes downward. • Dorsiflexion: Point toes upward. *Comments:*	☐	☐	☐	
k. *Foot (Gliding Joint)* • Eversion: Turn sole of foot laterally. • Inversion: Turn sole of foot medially. *Comments:*	☐	☐	☐	

Procedure 29-10	Able to Perform	Able to Perform with Assistance	Unable to Perform	Initials and Date
l. *Toes (Condyloid)* • Flexion: Curve toes downward. • Extension: Straighten toes. • Abduction: Spread toes apart. • Adduction: Bring toes together. *Comments:*	☐	☐	☐	
9. Observe client's joints and face for signs of exertion, pain, or fatigue during movement. *Comments:*	☐	☐	☐	
10. Replace covers and position client in proper body alignment. *Comments:*	☐	☐	☐	
11. Place side rails in original position. *Comments:*	☐	☐	☐	
12. Place call light within reach. *Comments:*	☐	☐	☐	
12. Wash hands. *Comments:*	☐	☐	☐	
Evaluation				
1. Client has maintained or improved current functional mobility in all involved joints and extremities. *Comments:*	☐	☐	☐	
2. Client has regained or improved strength and/or voluntary movement in involved joints and extremities. *Comments:*	☐	☐	☐	
3. Client has avoided complications of immobility, including pressure ulcers, contractures, decreased peristalsis, constipation, fecal impaction, orthostatic hypotension, pulmonary embolism, and thrombophlebitis. *Comments:*	☐	☐	☐	

Checklist for Procedure 29-11   Ambulation Safety and Assisting from Bed to Walking

Name _____ Date _____

School _____

Instructor _____

Course _____

Procedure 29-11 Ambulation Safety and Assisting from Bed to Walking	Able to Perform	Able to Perform with Assistance	Unable to Perform	Initials and Date
Assessment				
1. Determine the client's most recent activity level and tolerance to evaluate the client's current ambulatory ability. Comments:	☐	☐	☐	
2. Assess the client's current status, including vital signs, fatigue, pain, and medications, to identify conditions that might adversely affect ambulation. Comments:	☐	☐	☐	
3. To evaluate the client's environment for safety: Check for handrails to help client stand and to hold onto while walking. Check that the floor is level, clean, and not slippery or wet. Make sure there is adequate lighting so the client can see where he or she is going. Comments:	☐	☐	☐	
4. Assess the client's ambulation equipment, including the use of a walker, cane, or other assistive device to determine whether the equipment is in safe condition. Comments:	☐	☐	☐	
5. Check the client's clothing to determine that the client's shoes or slippers are safe to walk in and that he or she has adequate covering for warmth and privacy. Comments:	☐	☐	☐	
6. While the client is ambulating, assess his or her gait and bearing. Determines how well he or she is tolerating the activity and allows detection of hypotension, diaphoresis, breathlessness, or weakness. Comments:	☐	☐	☐	
7. After ambulation, assess the client's ability to recover from the activity, including exhaustion, energy, and recovery times. Determine if modifications need to be made in the distance, type of assistance, or length of time the client is ambulating. Comments:	☐	☐	☐	

continued on the following page

continued from the previous page

Procedure 29-11	Able to Perform	Able to Perform with Assistance	Unable to Perform	Initials and Date
Planning/Expected Outcomes				
1. The client will be able to walk a predetermined distance, with assistance as needed, and return to the starting point. *Comments:*	☐	☐	☐	
2. While walking, the client will not suffer any injury. *Comments:*	☐	☐	☐	
3. The client will be able to increase the distance he or she can walk and/or will require less assistance to accomplish the distance on a regular basis. *Comments:*	☐	☐	☐	
Implementation				
1. Wash hands, check client's identification band, and explain procedure before beginning. When assisting a client with an intravenous (IV) infusion, place the IV pole with wheels at the head of the bed before having the client dangle the legs, so there is room to swing the legs from the bed to the floor. If orders allow, place a saline lock on the IV. *Comments:*	☐	☐	☐	
2. If the facility does not maintain IVs on IV poles, transfer the IV infusion from the bed IV pole to the portable IV pole. The client or nurse can guide the portable IV pole ahead during ambulation. *Comments:*	☐	☐	☐	
3. When assisting the client with a urinary drainage bag, empty the drainage bag before ambulation. Have the client sit on the side of the bed with legs dangling. Remove the urinary drainage bag from the bed. The nurse or client can hold the urinary drainage bag during ambulation. Make sure the drainage bag remains below the level of the bladder. *Comments:*	☐	☐	☐	
4. When the client has a drainage tube, such as a T-tube, hemovac, or Jackson-Pratt drainage system, be sure to secure the drainage tube and bag before ambulation. Place a rubber band around the drainage tube near the drainage bag. Secure the drainage bag tube and bag with a safety pin through the rubber band. Allow slack. The safety pin is secured to the client's gown or robe. Make sure the safety pin is unfastened after the walk, so the tubing is not accidentally pulled when removing the gown. *Comments:*	☐	☐	☐	

Procedure 29-11	Able to Perform	Able to Perform with Assistance	Unable to Perform	Initials and Date
5. Ambulating the client with a closed chest tube drainage system often requires two nurses, one assisting the client and one nurse managing the closed chest tube drainage system. While the client is sitting on the edge of the bed with feet dangling, remove the hangers from the drainage system. Hold the closed chest tube drainage system upright at all times. Handle all IVs, tubes, and chest tubes gently so as not to dislodge any drains. *Comments:*	☐	☐	☐	
6. Use a transfer belt or gait belt when ambulating a client who is weak. For additional safety, a wheelchair can be pushed along behind the client for ready access if the client feels weak, tired, or faint. *Comments:*	☐	☐	☐	
7. If a client feels faint or dizzy during dangling, return the client to a supine position in bed and lower the head of the bed. Monitor the client's blood pressure and pulse. *Comments:*	☐	☐	☐	
8. If the client feels faint or dizzy during ambulation, allow the client to sit in a chair. Stay with the client for safety. Request another nurse to secure a wheelchair if not already available to return the client to bed. *Comments:*	☐	☐	☐	
9. If the client feels faint or dizzy during the ambulation and starts to fall, ease the client to the floor while supporting and protecting the client's head. Position yourself next to and slightly behind the ambulating client, so you are able to step behind the client and safely ease the client to the floor. Ask other personnel to assist you in returning the client to bed. Assess orthostatic blood pressure measurements. *Comments:*	☐	☐	☐	
10. Encourage the client to void before ambulating (especially an elderly client). *Comments:*	☐	☐	☐	
Bed to Walking				
1. Inform client of the purposes and distance of the walking exercise. *Comments:*	☐	☐	☐	

continued on the following page

continued from the previous page

Procedure 29-11	Able to Perform	Able to Perform with Assistance	Unable to Perform	Initials and Date
2. Elevate the head of the bed and wait several minutes. *Comments:*	☐	☐	☐	
3. Lower the bed height. *Comments:*	☐	☐	☐	
4. Encourage the client to actively move legs, or this may be done passively. *Comments:*	☐	☐	☐	
5. With one arm on the client's back and one arm under the client's upper legs, move the client into the dangling position. *Comments:*	☐	☐	☐	
6. Encourage the client to dangle at the side of the bed for several minutes. *Comments:*	☐	☐	☐	
7. Place gait belt around client's waist; secure the buckle in front. Place ambulation device such as a walker within reach of the client, if necessary. Assist the client into standing position. Make sure bed is locked and floor is not slippery. Client shoes should have nonslip soles. *Comments:*	☐	☐	☐	
8. Stand in front of client with your knees touching client's knees. *Comments:*	☐	☐	☐	
9. Place arms under client's axilla. *Comments:*	☐	☐	☐	
10. Assist client to a standing position, allowing client time to balance. *Comments:*	☐	☐	☐	
11. If the client is able to proceed with ambulating, assume a position beside the client and assist the client as necessary using the gait belt. Place yourself in a guarding position so as to assist client quickly and safely, if necessary. Use additional assistance as necessary. *Comments:*	☐	☐	☐	

Procedure 29-11	Able to Perform	Able to Perform with Assistance	Unable to Perform	Initials and Date
12. Following ambulation, return the client to bed, remove gait belt, and monitor vital signs, as necessary. Make the client comfortable and make sure all lines and tubes are secure. *Comments:*	☐	☐	☐	
13. Place call light within reach of the client. *Comments:*	☐	☐	☐	
14. Move the bedside table close to the bed and place items of frequent use within reach of the client. *Comments:*	☐	☐	☐	
15. Wash hands. *Comments:*	☐	☐	☐	
Evaluation				
1. The client was able to walk predetermined distance, with assistance as needed, and return to the starting point. *Comments:*	☐	☐	☐	
2. While walking, the client did not sustain any injury. *Comments:*	☐	☐	☐	
3. The client was able to increase the distance walked and/or required less assistance to accomplish the distance on a regular basis. *Comments:*	☐	☐	☐	

Checklist for Procedure 29-12   Assisting with Crutches, Cane, or Walker

Name _____   Date _____

School _____

Instructor _____

Course _____

Procedure 29-12 Assisting with Crutches, Cane, or Walker	Able to Perform	Able to Perform with Assistance	Unable to Perform	Initials and Date
Assessment				
1. Assess the reason the client requires an assistive device. Comments:	☐	☐	☐	
2. Assess the client's physical limitations. Comments:	☐	☐	☐	
3. Assess the client's physical environment. Comments:	☐	☐	☐	
4. Assess the client's ability to understand and follow directions. Comments:	☐	☐	☐	
Planning/Expected Outcomes				
1. The client will be able to demonstrate safe and independent ambulation with the assistance of crutches, a cane, or a walker.. Comments:	☐	☐	☐	
2. The client will feel confident and safe while using the assistive device. Comments:	☐	☐	☐	
Implementation				
Crutch Walking				
1. Check client's identification band and explain procedure before beginning. Assess the client for strength, mobility, range of motion, visual acuity, perceptual difficulties, and balance. Comments:	☐	☐	☐	
2. Adjust crutches to fit the client. Measure client for size of crutches and adjust crutches to fit. While client is supine, measure client from heel to axilla. When client is standing, the crutch pad should fit 1.5–2 inches below the axilla. Adjust hand grip so elbow is at 30-degree flexion. Comments:	☐	☐	☐	

continued on the following page

continued from the previous page

Procedure 29-12	Able to Perform	Able to Perform with Assistance	Unable to Perform	Initials and Date
3. Provide a robe or other covering as well as nonslip foot coverings or shoes. *Comments:*	☐	☐	☐	
4. Lower the height of the bed. *Comments:*	☐	☐	☐	
5. Dangle the client at the side of the bed for several minutes. Assess for vertigo or nausea. *Comments:*	☐	☐	☐	
6. Apply the gait belt around the client's waist if balance and stability are unknown or unreliable. *Comments:*	☐	☐	☐	
7. Demonstrate to client the method of holding crutches while he or she remains seated. This should be with elbows bent 30 degrees while hands are on the handgrips and pads 1.5–2 inches below the axilla. Instruct client to position crutches 4–5 inches laterally and 4–6 inches in front of feet, with weight on hands, not axilla. *Comments:*	☐	☐	☐	
8. Assist the client to a standing position by having client place both crutches in nondominent hand. Then, using the dominant hand, client can push off from the bed while using the crutches for balance. Once erect, the extra crutch can be moved into the dominant hand. *Comments:*	☐	☐	☐	
9. Instruct the client to remain still for a few seconds while assessing for vertigo or nausea. Stand close to the client to support as needed. While client remains standing, check for correct fit of the crutches. *Comments:*	☐	☐	☐	
Two-Point Gait 10. • Move the left crutch and right leg forward 4–6 inches. • Move the right crutch and left leg forward 4–6 inches. • Repeat the two-point gait. *Comments:*	☐	☐	☐	

Procedure 29-12	Able to Perform	Able to Perform with Assistance	Unable to Perform	Initials and Date
Three-Point Gait				
11. • Advance both crutches and the weaker leg forward together 4–6 inches. • Move the stronger leg forward, even with the crutches. • Repeat the three-point gait. *Comments:*	☐	☐	☐	
Four-Point Gait				
12. • Position crutches 4.5–6 inches to the side and in front of each foot. • Move the right crutch forward 4–6 inches. • Move the left foot forward, even with the left crutch. • Move the left crutch forward 4–6 inches. • Move the right foot forward, even with the right crutch. • Repeat the four-point gait. *Comments:*	☐	☐	☐	
Swing-Through Gait				
13. • Move both crutches forward together 4–6 inches. • Move both legs forward in a swinging motion past the crutches. • Repeat the swing-through gait. *Comments:*	☐	☐	☐	
Walking Up Stairs				
14. • Stand beside and slightly behind the client. Instruct the client to position the crutches as if walking. Place body weight on hands. • Place the strong leg on the first step. • Pull the weak leg up and move the crutches up to the first step. • Repeat for all steps. *Comments:*	☐	☐	☐	
Walking Down Stairs				
15. • Position the crutches as if walking. • Place weight on the strong leg. • Move the crutches down to the next lower step. • Place partial weight on hands and crutches. • Move the weak leg down to the step with the crutches. • Put total weight on arms and crutches. • Move strong leg to same step as weak leg and crutches. • Repeat for all steps. • A second caregiver standing behind the client holding onto the gait belt will further decrease the risk of falling. *Comments:*	☐	☐	☐	

continued on the following page

continued from the previous page

Procedure 29-12	Able to Perform	Able to Perform with Assistance	Unable to Perform	Initials and Date
16. Set realistic goals and opportunities for progressive ambulation using crutches. *Comments:*	☐	☐	☐	
17. Consult with a physical therapist for clients learning to walk with crutches. *Comments:*	☐	☐	☐	
18. Wash hands. *Comments:*	☐	☐	☐	
Sitting with Crutches				
19. Instruct the client to back up to chair until it is felt with the back of the legs. *Comments:*	☐	☐	☐	
20. Place both crutches in the nondominant hand and use the dominant hand to reach back to the chair. *Comments:*	☐	☐	☐	
21. Instruct the client to lower slowly into the chair. *Comments:*	☐	☐	☐	
Walking with a Cane				
22. Repeat Actions 1–6. *Comments:*	☐	☐	☐	
23. Have the client push up from the sitting position while pushing down on the bed with arms. *Comments:*	☐	☐	☐	
24. Have the client stand at the bedside for a few moments with cane in hand opposite the affected leg. *Comments:*	☐	☐	☐	
25. Assess the height of the cane. With the cane placed 6 inches ahead of the client's body, the top of the cane should be at wrist level with the arm bent 25%–30% at the elbow. *Comments:*	☐	☐	☐	

Procedure 29-12	Able to Perform	Able to Perform with Assistance	Unable to Perform	Initials and Date
26. Walk to the side and slightly behind the client, holding the gait belt if needed for stability. *Comments:*	☐	☐	☐	
The Cane Gait				
27. • Move the cane and the weaker leg forward at the same time for the same distance. • Place weight on the weaker leg and the cane. • Move the strong leg forward. • Place weight on the strong leg. *Comments:*	☐	☐	☐	
Sitting with a Cane				
28. • Have the client turn around and back up to the chair. • Have client grasp the arm of the chair with the free hand and lower self into the chair. • Be sure to place the cane out of the way but within reach. *Comments:*	☐	☐	☐	
29. Consult with a physical therapist for client's learning to walk with a cane. *Comments:*	☐	☐	☐	
30. Wash hands. *Comments:*	☐	☐	☐	
Walking with a Walker				
31. Repeat Actions 1–6. *Comments:*	☐	☐	☐	
32. Place the walker in front of the client. *Comments:*	☐	☐	☐	
33. Have the client put the nondominant hand on the front bar of the walker or on the handgrip for that hand, whichever is more comfortable. Then, with client using the dominant hand to push off from the bed and the nondominant hand for stabilization, help the client to an erect position. *Comments:*	☐	☐	☐	
34. Have the client transfer hand to the walker handgrips. *Comments:*	☐	☐	☐	

continued on the following page

continued from the previous page

Procedure 29-12	Able to Perform	Able to Perform with Assistance	Unable to Perform	Initials and Date
35. Be sure the walker is adjusted so the handgrips are just below waist level and the client's arms are slightly bent at the elbow. *Comments:*	☐	☐	☐	
36. Walk to the side and slightly behind the client, holding the gait belt if needed for stability. *Comments:*	☐	☐	☐	
The Walker Gait				
37. • Move the walker and weaker leg forward at the same time. • Place as much weight as possible or as allowed on the weaker leg, using the arms for supporting the rest of the weight. • Move the strong leg forward and shift the weight to the strong leg. *Comments:*	☐	☐	☐	
Sitting with a Walker				
38. • Have the client turn around in front of the chair and back up until the back of the legs touch the chair. • Have the client place hands on the chair armrests, one hand at a time, then lower self into chair using the armrests for support. *Comments:*	☐	☐	☐	
39. Consult with a physical therapist for clients learning to walk with a walker. *Comments:*	☐	☐	☐	
40. Wash hands. *Comments:*	☐	☐	☐	
Evaluation				
1. The client is able to demonstrate safe and independent ambulation with the assistance of crutches, a cane, or a walker. *Comments:*	☐	☐	☐	
2. The client feels confident and safe while using the assistive device. *Comments:*	☐	☐	☐	

Checklist for Procedure 29-13   Turning and Positioning a Client

Name _____   Date _____

School _____

Instructor _____

Course _____

Procedure 29-13 Turning and Positioning a Client	Able to Perform	Able to Perform with Assistance	Unable to Perform	Initials and Date
Assessment				
1. Assess the client's ability to move independently. Determine if the client can assist with turning and repositioning. *Comments:*	☐	☐	☐	
2. Assess the client's flexibility. *Comments:*	☐	☐	☐	
3. Assess the client's age, medical diagnosis, cognitive status, skin integrity, nutritional status, continence, altered sensation, as well as the overall condition of the musculoskeletal system. *Comments:*	☐	☐	☐	
4. Assess the physician's or qualified practitioner's orders for specific restrictions regarding client positioning. *Comments:*	☐	☐	☐	
Planning/Expected Outcomes				
1. The client will maintain skin integrity without skin burns, pressure areas, or pressure ulcers. *Comments:*	☐	☐	☐	
2. The client will be comfortable, as evidenced by verbal and nonverbal cues. *Comments:*	☐	☐	☐	
Implementation				
1. Wash hands, check client's identification band, and explain procedure before beginning. *Comments:*	☐	☐	☐	
2. Gather all necessary equipment. Provide for client privacy. *Comments:*	☐	☐	☐	

continued on the following page

continued from the previous page

Procedure 29-13	Able to Perform	Able to Perform with Assistance	Unable to Perform	Initials and Date
3. Secure adequate assistance to safely complete task. *Comments:*	☐	☐	☐	
4. Adjust bed to comfortable working height. Lower side rail on side of bed from which you are assisting client. *Comments:*	☐	☐	☐	
5. Follow proper body mechanics guidelines. *Comments:*	☐	☐	☐	
6. Position drains, tubes, and IVs to accommodate new client position. *Comments:*	☐	☐	☐	
7. Place or assist client into appropriate starting position. Monitor client status, and provide adequate rest breaks or support as necessary. *Comments:*	☐	☐	☐	
Moving from Supine to Side-Lying Position				
8. Move the client to one side of the bed by lifting the client's body toward you. Roll the client to side-lying position. *Comments:*	☐	☐	☐	
Maintaining Side-Lying Position				
9. Follow Actions 1–8. *Comments:*	☐	☐	☐	
10. Pillows may be placed to support the client. *Comments:*	☐	☐	☐	
Moving from Side-Lying to Prone Position				
11. Repeat Actions 1–8. *Comments:*	☐	☐	☐	
12. Remove positioning support devices. Move the client's inside arm next to the client's body. Roll the client onto the stomach. Place pillows as needed. *Comments:*	☐	☐	☐	

Procedure 29-13	Able to Perform	Able to Perform with Assistance	Unable to Perform	Initials and Date
Maintaining Prone Position				
13. Pillows or a folded towel may be used to support the client. *Comments:*	☐	☐	☐	
Moving from Prone to Supine Position				
14. Repeat Actions 1–8. *Comments:*	☐	☐	☐	
15. Remove supporting devices. Move the client to one side of the bed. Log roll the client toward you. *Comments:*	☐	☐	☐	
Maintaining the Supine Position				
16. Pillows, a footboard, heel protectors, or a trochanter roll may be used to support the client. *Comments:*	☐	☐	☐	
Log Rolling				
17. Repeat Actions 1–8. *Comments:*	☐	☐	☐	
18. Use three nurses. Place a turn/draw sheet under client's head, back, and buttocks (if not already present). *Comments:*	☐	☐	☐	
19. Place a pillow between the client's legs. *Comments:*	☐	☐	☐	
20. Have the client fold arms across the chest. *Comments:*	☐	☐	☐	
21. Roll up draw sheet on the far side until it is next to the client. *Comments:*	☐	☐	☐	
22. One nurse places hands under the client's far leg, another holds a rolled draw sheet at the client's buttocks, and a third nurse holds a rolled draw sheet at chest and shoulder level. *Comments:*	☐	☐	☐	

continued on the following page

continued from the previous page

Procedure 29-13	Able to Perform	Able to Perform with Assistance	Unable to Perform	Initials and Date
23. Nurse nearest the client's head gives the signal to turn: 1–2–3 turn. *Comments:*	☐	☐	☐	
24. Tuck pillows at client's back and abdomen. *Comments:*	☐	☐	☐	
25. Assess the client for comfort and proper alignment. *Comments:*	☐	☐	☐	
26. Procedure can be reversed to reposition client on back or opposite side. *Comments:*	☐	☐	☐	
27. Replace side rails to upright position and lower the bed. *Comments:*	☐	☐	☐	
28. Place call light within reach of the client. *Comments:*	☐	☐	☐	
29. Move bedside table close to bed and place items of frequent use within reach of the client. *Comments:*	☐	☐	☐	
30. Wash hands. *Comments:*	☐	☐	☐	

Evaluation

	Able to Perform	Able to Perform with Assistance	Unable to Perform	Initials and Date
1. Safe and proper body alignment and movement were achieved for both the client and caregiver. *Comments:*	☐	☐	☐	
2. The client is comfortable in the new position, as evident from verbal and nonverbal cues. *Comments:*	☐	☐	☐	
3. The client's skin and underlying organs and tissues were protected from pressure, friction, and shear. *Comments:*	☐	☐	☐	

Checklist for Procedure 29-14   Moving a Client in Bed

Name _____   Date _____

School _____

Instructor _____

Course _____

Procedure 29-14 Moving a Client in Bed	Able to Perform	Able to Perform with Assistance	Unable to Perform	Initials and Date
Assessment				
1. Assess the client's ability to assist with repositioning. Determine whether the client can move with the aid of an overhead trapeze or the side rail. Judge how much assistance will be needed. *Comments:*	☐	☐	☐	
2. Assess the client's ability to understand and follow directions and assist and cooperate with the move. *Comments:*	☐	☐	☐	
3. Assess the client's environment and bed for cleanliness. Has the client been restless, sweaty, or incontinent? Check to see if the sheets are turned or twisted. Tubes, lines, wires, traction, casts, or splints are moved carefully. Affects how the procedure is completed. *Comments:*	☐	☐	☐	
Planning/Expected Outcomes				
1. The client will be moved in bed without injury to self. *Comments:*	☐	☐	☐	
2. The client will be moved in bed without injury to the staff. *Comments:*	☐	☐	☐	
3. The client will report an increase in comfort following the move. *Comments:*	☐	☐	☐	
4. All tubes, lines, and drains will remain patent and intact. *Comments:*	☐	☐	☐	

continued on the following page

continued from the previous page

Procedure 29-14	Able to Perform	Able to Perform with Assistance	Unable to Perform	Initials and Date
Implementation				
Moving a Client Up in Bed with One Nurse				
1. Wash hands, check client's identification band, and explain procedure before beginning. *Comments:*	☐	☐	☐	
2. Elevate bed to just below waist height. Lower head of bed if tolerated by client. Lower side rails on the side where you are standing. *Comments:*	☐	☐	☐	
3. Place the pillow against the headboard. *Comments:*	☐	☐	☐	
4. Have client hold onto the overhead trapeze, if available. *Comments:*	☐	☐	☐	
5. Have the client bend knees and place feet flat on the bed if able. *Comments:*	☐	☐	☐	
6. Stand at an angle to the head of the bed, feet apart, knees bent, and feet toward the head of the bed. *Comments:*	☐	☐	☐	
7. Slide one hand and arm under the client's shoulder, the other under the client's thigh. *Comments:*	☐	☐	☐	
8. Rock forward toward the head of the bed, lifting the client with you. Simultaneously have the client push with the legs. *Comments:*	☐	☐	☐	
9. If the client has a trapeze, have the client pull up, holding onto the trapeze, as you move the client upward in bed. *Comments:*	☐	☐	☐	
10. Repeat these steps until the client is moved up high enough in bed. *Comments:*	☐	☐	☐	

Procedure 29-14	Able to Perform	Able to Perform with Assistance	Unable to Perform	Initials and Date
11. Return the client's pillow under the head. *Comments:*	☐	☐	☐	
12. Elevate the head of bed, if tolerated by the client. *Comments:*	☐	☐	☐	
13. Assess the client for comfort. *Comments:*	☐	☐	☐	
14. Adjust the client's bedclothes as needed for comfort. *Comments:*	☐	☐	☐	
15. Lower bed and elevate side rails. *Comments:*	☐	☐	☐	
16. Wash hands. *Comments:*	☐	☐	☐	
Moving a Client Up in Bed with Two or More Nurses				
17. Wash hands and apply gloves if needed. *Comments:*	☐	☐	☐	
18. Elevate bed to just below waist height. Lower head of bed if tolerated by client. Lower side rails. *Comments:*	☐	☐	☐	
19. With two nurses, place a turn/draw sheet under the client's back and head. *Comments:*	☐	☐	☐	
20. Roll up the draw sheet on each side until it is next to the client. *Comments:*	☐	☐	☐	
21. Follow previous Actions 3–5. *Comments:*	☐	☐	☐	
22. The nurses stand on either side of the bed, at an angle to the head of the bed, with knees flexed, feet apart in a wide stance. *Comments:*	☐	☐	☐	

continued on the following page

continued from the previous page

Procedure 29-14	**Able to Perform**	**Able to Perform with Assistance**	**Unable to Perform**	**Initials and Date**
23. The nurses hold their elbows as close as possible to their bodies. *Comments:*	☐	☐	☐	
24. The lead nurse gives the signal to move: 1–2–3 go. The nurses lift the turn/draw sheet off the bed and toward the head of the bed in one smooth motion. Simultaneously, the client pushes with the legs or pulls using the trapeze. *Comments:*	☐	☐	☐	
25. Repeat previous Actions 10–16. *Comments:*	☐	☐	☐	
Evaluation				
1. The client was moved without injury to self or staff. *Comments:*	☐	☐	☐	
2. The client reported an increase in comfort following the move. *Comments:*	☐	☐	☐	
3. All tubes, lines, and drains remained intact. *Comments:*	☐	☐	☐	

Checklist for Procedure 29-15   Transferring from Bed to Wheelchair, Commode, or Chair

Name _____ Date _____

School _____

Instructor _____

Course _____

Procedure 29-15 Transferring from Bed to Wheelchair, Commode, or Chair	Able to Perform	Able to Perform with Assistance	Unable to Perform	Initials and Date
Assessment				
1. Assess the client's current level of mobility. Determine how much the client is able to assist with the transfer. Assess for pain or confusion, which might impair ability to assist. Check for a "weak" side. *Comments:*	☐	☐	☐	
2. Assess for any impediments to mobility, including casts, drainage tubes, catheters, IVs, or intubation. *Comments:*	☐	☐	☐	
3. Assess the client's level of understanding and anxiety regarding the procedure. *Comments:*	☐	☐	☐	
4. Assess the client's environment. *Comments:*	☐	☐	☐	
5. Assess the equipment. *Comments:*	☐	☐	☐	
Planning/Expected Outcomes				
1. The client will be transferred from the bed to the wheelchair, commode, or chair without pain or injury. *Comments:*	☐	☐	☐	
2. Drainage tubes, IVs, or other devices will be intact. *Comments:*	☐	☐	☐	
3. The client's skin will be intact and undamaged. *Comments:*	☐	☐	☐	
Implementation				
1. Wash hands, check client's identification band, and explain procedure before beginning. *Comments:*	☐	☐	☐	

continued on the following page

continued from the previous page

Procedure 29-15	Able to Perform	Able to Perform with Assistance	Unable to Perform	Initials and Date
2. Assess client for ability to assist with the transfer and for presence of cognitive or sensory deficits. *Comments:*	☐	☐	☐	
3. Lock the bed in position. *Comments:*	☐	☐	☐	
4. Place any splints, braces, or other devices on the client. *Comments:*	☐	☐	☐	
5. Place the client's shoes or slippers on the client's feet. *Comments:*	☐	☐	☐	
6. Lower the height of the bed to the lowest possible position. *Comments:*	☐	☐	☐	
7. Slowly raise the head of the bed if this is not contraindicated by the client's condition. *Comments:*	☐	☐	☐	
8. Place one arm under the client's legs and one arm behind the client's back. Slowly pivot the client so the client's legs are dangling over the edge of the bed and the client is in a sitting position on the edge of the bed. *Comments:*	☐	☐	☐	
9. Allow the client to dangle for 2–5 minutes. Help support client if necessary. *Comments:*	☐	☐	☐	
10. Bring the chair or wheelchair close to the side of the bed. Place it at a 45-degree angle to the bed. If the client has a weaker side, place the chair or wheelchair on the client's strong side. *Comments:*	☐	☐	☐	
11. Lock wheelchair brakes and elevate the foot pedals. For chairs, lock brakes if available. *Comments:*	☐	☐	☐	
12. If using a gait belt to assist the client, place it around the client's waist. *Comments:*	☐	☐	☐	

Procedure 29-15	Able to Perform	Able to Perform with Assistance	Unable to Perform	Initials and Date
13. Assist client to side of the bed until feet are firmly on the floor and slightly apart. *Comments:*	☐	☐	☐	
14. Grasp the sides of the gait belt or place your hands just below the client's axilla. Using a wide stance, bend your knees and assist the client to a standing position. *Comments:*	☐	☐	☐	
15. Standing close to the client, pivot until the client's back is toward the chair. *Comments:*	☐	☐	☐	
16. Instruct the client to place hands on the arm supports, or place the client's hands on the supports of the chair. *Comments:*	☐	☐	☐	
17. Bend at the knees and ease the client into a sitting position. *Comments:*	☐	☐	☐	
18. Assist client to maintain proper posture. Support weak side with pillow if needed. *Comments:*	☐	☐	☐	
19. Secure the safety belt, place client's feet on foot pedals, and release brakes if you will be moving the client immediately. Make sure tubes and lines, arms, and hands are not pinched or caught between the client and the chair. If a client is sitting in a wheelchair, position the footrests in a position of client comfort; if in a chair, offer a footstool if available. *Comments:*	☐	☐	☐	
20. Wash hands. *Comments:*	☐	☐	☐	
Evaluation				
1. Client was transferred from the bed to the wheelchair without pain or injury. *Comments:*	☐	☐	☐	

continued on the following page

continued from the previous page

Procedure 29-15	Able to Perform	Able to Perform with Assistance	Unable to Perform	Initials and Date
2. Drainage tubes, IVs, or other devices remain intact. *Comments:*	☐	☐	☐	
3. Client's skin is intact and undamaged. *Comments:*	☐	☐	☐	

Checklist for Procedure 29-16   Transferring from Bed to Stretcher

Name _____ Date _____

School _____

Instructor _____

Course _____

Procedure 29-16 Transferring from Bed to Stretcher	Able to Perform	Able to Perform with Assistance	Unable to Perform	Initials and Date
Assessment				
1. Assess the client's current level of mobility. *Comments:*	☐	☐	☐	
2. Assess for injury. *Comments:*	☐	☐	☐	
3. Assess for any impediments to mobility, such as a cast, drainage tubes, IVs, or intubation. *Comments:*	☐	☐	☐	
4. Assess the client's level of understanding of the procedure. *Comments:*	☐	☐	☐	
5. Assess the client's environment. Assess how close the stretcher will move to the bed and the height of the bed. Plan for good body mechanics. *Comments:*	☐	☐	☐	
6. Make sure the stretcher is safe to use. Check that working brakes, side rails, and safety straps are intact and usable, and that there is an IV pole attachment if needed. Plan for good body mechanics *Comments:*	☐	☐	☐	
Planning/Expected Outcomes				
1. The client will be transferred from the bed to the stretcher without pain or injury. *Comments:*	☐	☐	☐	
2. Drainage tubes, IVs, or other devices will remain intact. *Comments:*	☐	☐	☐	
3. The client's skin will be intact and undamaged. *Comments:*	☐	☐	☐	

continued on the following page

continued from the previous page

Procedure 29-16	Able to Perform	Able to Perform with Assistance	Unable to Perform	Initials and Date
Implementation				
Transferring a Client with Minimum Assistance				
1. Wash hands, check client's identification band, and explain procedure before beginning. *Comments:*	☐	☐	☐	
2. Raise the height of bed 1 inch higher than the stretcher and lock brakes of bed. *Comments:*	☐	☐	☐	
3. Instruct client to move to side of bed close to the stretcher. Lower side rails of bed and stretcher. Leave side rails on opposite side up. *Comments:*	☐	☐	☐	
4. Stand at outer side of stretcher and push it toward bed. *Comments:*	☐	☐	☐	
5. Instruct client to move onto stretcher with assistance as needed. *Comments:*	☐	☐	☐	
6. Cover client with sheet or bath blanket. *Comments:*	☐	☐	☐	
7. Elevate side rails on stretcher and secure safety belts about client. Release brakes of stretcher. *Comments:*	☐	☐	☐	
8. Stand at head of stretcher to guide it when pushing. *Comments:*	☐	☐	☐	
9. Wash hands. *Comments:*	☐	☐	☐	
Transferring a Client with Maximum Assistance				
10. Repeat Actions 1 and 2. *Comments:*	☐	☐	☐	
11. Assess amount of assistance required for transfer. *Comments:*	☐	☐	☐	

Procedure 29-16	Able to Perform	Able to Perform with Assistance	Unable to Perform	Initials and Date
12. Lock wheels of bed and stretcher. *Comments:*	☐	☐	☐	
13. Have one nurse stand close to the client's head. *Comments:*	☐	☐	☐	
14. Log roll the client (keep in straight alignment) and place a lift sheet under the client's back, trunk, and upper legs. The lift sheet can extend under the head if client lacks head control abilities. *Comments:*	☐	☐	☐	
15. Empty all drainage bags. Record amounts. Secure drainage system to the client's gown before transfer. *Comments:*	☐	☐	☐	
16. Move client to edge of bed near stretcher. Lift up and over to avoid dragging. *Comments:*	☐	☐	☐	
17. The nurse on the nonstretcher side of the bed holds the stretcher side of the lift sheet up to prevent the client from falling. *Comments:*	☐	☐	☐	
18. Place pillow and slider board overlapping the bed and stretcher. *Comments:*	☐	☐	☐	
19. Have staff members grasp edges of lift sheet. Be sure to use good body mechanics. *Comments:*	☐	☐	☐	
20. On the count of three, have staff members pull lift sheet and the client onto the stretcher. *Comments:*	☐	☐	☐	
21. Position the client on stretcher, place pillow under head, and cover with a sheet or bath blanket. *Comments:*	☐	☐	☐	

continued on the following page

continued from the previous page

Procedure 29-16	Able to Perform	Able to Perform with Assistance	Unable to Perform	Initials and Date
22. Secure safety belts and elevate side rails of stretcher. *Comments:*	☐	☐	☐	
23. If IV is present, move it from bed IV pole to stretcher IV pole after client transfer. *Comments:*	☐	☐	☐	
24. Wash hands. *Comments:*	☐	☐	☐	
Evaluation				
1. Client was transferred from the bed to the stretcher without pain or injury. *Comments:*	☐	☐	☐	
2. All drainage tubes, IVs, or other devices remained intact. *Comments:*	☐	☐	☐	
3. Client's skin remained intact and undamaged. *Comments:*	☐	☐	☐	

Checklist for Procedure 29-17   Bedmaking: Unoccupied Bed

Name _____ Date _____

School _____

Instructor _____

Course _____

Procedure 29-17 Bedmaking: Unoccupied Bed	Able to Perform	Able to Perform with Assistance	Unable to Perform	Initials and Date
Assessment				
1. Assess your equipment. Check for all linens necessary to change the bed. Check for a dirty linen hamper. *Comments:*	☐	☐	☐	
2. Assess whether the bed itself needs cleaning before placing clean sheet on it. *Comments:*	☐	☐	☐	
3. Assess the client's needs in the bed. Check for profuse drainage, incontinence, or special needs for comfort or skin integrity. *Comments:*	☐	☐	☐	
4. Assess the client's ability to be out of bed in a safe place while changing linens. *Comments:*	☐	☐	☐	
Planning/Expected Outcomes				
1. The client will have clean linens on the bed. *Comments:*	☐	☐	☐	
2. The clean linens will be appropriate to the client's needs and condition. *Comments:*	☐	☐	☐	
Implementation				
Preparation 1. Wash hands, check client's identification band, and explain procedure before beginning. Place hamper by client's door if linen bags are not available. Assess condition of blankets and/or bedspread. *Comments:*	☐	☐	☐	

continued on the following page

continued from the previous page

Procedure 29-17	Able to Perform	Able to Perform with Assistance	Unable to Perform	Initials and Date
2. Gather linens and gloves. Places linens on a clean, dry surface in reverse order of usage at the client's bedside (pillowcases, top sheet, draw sheet, bottom sheet). *Comments:*	☐	☐	☐	
3. Inquire about the client's toileting needs and attend as necessary. *Comments:*	☐	☐	☐	
4. Assist client to a safe, comfortable chair. *Comments:*	☐	☐	☐	
5. Apply gloves. *Comments:*	☐	☐	☐	
6. Position bed: flat, side rails down, adjust height to waist level. *Comments:*	☐	☐	☐	
7. Remove and fold blanket and/or bedspread. If clean and reusable, place on clean work area. *Comments:*	☐	☐	☐	
8. Remove soiled pillowcases by grasping the closed end with one hand and slipping the pillow out with the other. Place the soiled cases on top of the soiled sheet, and place the pillows on clean work area. *Comments:*	☐	☐	☐	
9. Remove soiled linens: Start on the side of the bed closest to you; free the bottom sheet and mattress pad (if used) by lifting the mattress and rolling soiled linens to the middle of the bed. Go to the other side of the bed, repeat action. *Comments:*	☐	☐	☐	
10. Fold soiled linens (do not fan or flap): head of bed to middle, then foot of bed to middle. Place in linen bag, keeping soiled linens away from uniform. *Comments:*	☐	☐	☐	
11. Check the mattress and clean if needed. *Comments:*	☐	☐	☐	

Procedure 29-17	Able to Perform	Able to Perform with Assistance	Unable to Perform	Initials and Date
12. Remove gloves, cleanse hands, and apply a second pair of clean gloves. *Comments:*	☐	☐	☐	
13. Open the clean mattress pad lengthwise onto the bed. Unfold half of the pad's width to the center crease and smooth the pad flat. If there are elastic bands to hold the pad in place, slide them under the corners of the mattress. *Comments:*	☐	☐	☐	
14. Place bottom sheet onto the mattress. Linens differ from facility to facility. Bottom sheets may be fitted or flat. Proceed to the appropriate action for the linen available. *Comments:*	☐	☐	☐	
Fitted Bottom Sheet				
15. Position yourself diagonally toward the head of the bed. *Comments:*	☐	☐	☐	
16. Start at the head with seemed side of the fitted sheet toward the mattress. *Comments:*	☐	☐	☐	
17. Lift the mattress corner with your hand closest to the bed; with your other hand, pull and tuck the fitted sheet over the mattress corner; secure at the head of the bed. *Comments:*	☐	☐	☐	
18. Pull and tuck the fitted sheet over the mattress corners at the foot of the bed. *Comments:*	☐	☐	☐	
Flat Regular Sheet				
19. Unfold the bottom sheet with the seemed side toward the mattress. Align the bottom edge of the sheet with the edge of the mattress at the foot of the bed. *Comments:*	☐	☐	☐	
20. Allow the sheet to hang 10 inches (25 cm) over the mattress on the side and at the top of the bed. *Comments:*	☐	☐	☐	

continued on the following page

continued from the previous page

Procedure 29-17	Able to Perform	Able to Perform with Assistance	Unable to Perform	Initials and Date
21. Position yourself diagonally toward the head of the bed. Lift the top of the mattress corner with the hand closest to the bed and smoothly tuck the sheet under the mattress. *Comments:*	☐	☐	☐	
22. Miter the corner at the head of the bed. *Comments:*	☐	☐	☐	
23. Lift and lay the top edge of the sheet onto the bed to form a triangular fold. *Comments:*	☐	☐	☐	
24. Tuck the lower edge of the sheet under the mattress. *Comments:*	☐	☐	☐	
25. Bring the triangular fold down over the side of the mattress. *Comments:*	☐	☐	☐	
26. Place the draw sheet on the bottom sheet and unfold it to the middle crease. *Comments:*	☐	☐	☐	
27. Tuck both the bottom and draw sheets smoothly under the mattress. *Comments:*	☐	☐	☐	
28. On the other side of the bed, unfold the bottom sheet, and repeat the actions used to apply the mattress pad and bottom sheet. *Comments:*	☐	☐	☐	
29. Unfold the draw sheet, if used, and grasp the free-hanging sides of both the bottom and draw sheets. *Comments:*	☐	☐	☐	
30. Place the top sheet on the bed. Place the top edge of the sheet even with the top of the mattress. Pull the remaining length toward the bottom of the bed. *Comments:*	☐	☐	☐	

Procedure 29-17	Able to Perform	Able to Perform with Assistance	Unable to Perform	Initials and Date
31. Unfold and apply the blanket or spread. Follow the same technique as used in applying the top sheet. *Comments:*	☐	☐	☐	
32. Miter the bottom corners. *Comments:*	☐	☐	☐	
33. Fold the top sheet and blanket over. Fan-fold the sheet and blanket. *Comments:*	☐	☐	☐	
34. Apply a clean pillowcase on each pillow. With one hand, grasp the closed end of the pillowcase. Gather the pillowcase and turn it inside out over hand. With the same hand, grasp the middle of one end of the pillow. With the other hand, pull the case over the length of the pillow. *Comments:*	☐	☐	☐	
35. Return the bed to the lowest position and elevate the head of the bed 30–45 degrees. Put side rails up on side farthest from the client. *Comments:*	☐	☐	☐	
36. Inquire about the toileting needs of the client; assist as necessary. *Comments:*	☐	☐	☐	
37. Assist the client back into the bed and pull up the side rails; place call light in reach; take vital signs. *Comments:*	☐	☐	☐	
38. Remove gloves and wash hands. *Comments:*	☐	☐	☐	
Evaluation				
1. Confirm that fresh linens were placed on the bed in a manner appropriate to the client's needs. *Comments:*	☐	☐	☐	

Checklist for Procedure 29-18   Bedmaking: Occupied Bed

Name _____ Date _____

School _____

Instructor _____

Course _____

Procedure 29-18 Bedmaking: Occupied Bed	Able to Perform	Able to Perform with Assistance	Unable to Perform	Initials and Date
Assessment				
1. Assess your equipment. Check for all the linens necessary to change the bed. *Comments:*	☐	☐	☐	
2. Assess whether the bed itself needs cleaning before placing clean sheets on it. *Comments:*	☐	☐	☐	
3. Assess the client's needs in the bed. Check for profuse drainage, incontinence, or special needs for comfort or skin integrity. *Comments:*	☐	☐	☐	
4. Assess the client's ability to assist with the procedure, including mobility, mental status, and muscle strength. *Comments:*	☐	☐	☐	
5. Assess for the presence of dressings, IVs, tubes, or any equipment that may be attached to the client. *Comments:*	☐	☐	☐	
Planning/Expected Outcomes				
1. The client will have clean linens on the bed. *Comments:*	☐	☐	☐	
2. The clean linens will be appropriate to the client's needs and condition. *Comments:*	☐	☐	☐	
3. The linens will be changed with a minimum of trauma to the client. *Comments:*	☐	☐	☐	

continued on the following page

continued from the previous page

Procedure 29-18	Able to Perform	Able to Perform with Assistance	Unable to Perform	Initials and Date
Implementation				
1. Wash hands, check client's identification band, and explain procedure before beginning. *Comments:*	☐	☐	☐	
2. Bring equipment to the bedside. *Comments:*	☐	☐	☐	
3. Cover client with a bath blanket. Remove top sheet and blanket. Loosen bottom sheet at foot and sides of bed. *Comments:*	☐	☐	☐	
4. Position client on side, facing away from you. Reposition pillow under head. *Comments:*	☐	☐	☐	
5. Fan-fold or roll bottom linens close to client toward the center of the bed. *Comments:*	☐	☐	☐	
6. Place clean bottom linens with the center fold nearest the client. Fan-fold or roll clean bottom linens nearest client and tuck under soiled linen. If fitted sheets are not available, maintain an amount of sheet at head of bed for tucking. Have sheet even with bottom of mattress. *Comments:*	☐	☐	☐	
7. If fitted sheets are not available, miter bottom sheet at the head of the bed. Repeat for each corner. Tuck the sides of the sheet under the mattress. *Comments:*	☐	☐	☐	
8. Fan-fold or roll draw sheet and tuck under soiled linen. Tuck draw sheet under mattress. *Comments:*	☐	☐	☐	
9. Roll the client over onto side facing you. Raise side rail. *Comments:*	☐	☐	☐	
10. Move to the other side of bed. Remove soiled linens and place in linen bag without touching uniform. *Comments:*	☐	☐	☐	

Procedure 29-18	Able to Perform	Able to Perform with Assistance	Unable to Perform	Initials and Date
11. Unfold/unroll bottom sheet; then draw sheet. Look for objects left in the bed. Grasp each sheet with knuckles up and over the sheet, and pull tightly while leaning back with your body weight. Client may be positioned supine. Tuck in. *Comments:*	☐	☐	☐	
12. Place top sheet and blanket over the client. Remove bath blankets left on the client. *Comments:*	☐	☐	☐	
13. Raise foot of mattress and miter the corner. Repeat on other side. *Comments:*	☐	☐	☐	
14. Tent top sheet and blanket over the client's toes. *Comments:*	☐	☐	☐	
15. Remove soiled pillowcase and replace with clean pillowcase. *Comments:*	☐	☐	☐	
16. Wash hands. *Comments:*	☐	☐	☐	
Evaluation				
1. The client has clean, unwrinkled linen. *Comments:*	☐	☐	☐	
2. The linen placed on the bed is suitable for the client's special needs. *Comments:*	☐	☐	☐	
3. The linen was changed with a minimum of pain and trauma to the client. *Comments:*	☐	☐	☐	

Checklist for Procedure 29-19   Bathing a Client in Bed

Name _____   Date _____

School _____

Instructor _____

Course _____

Procedure 29-19 Bathing a Client in Bed	Able to Perform	Able to Perform with Assistance	Unable to Perform	Initials and Date
Assessment				
1. Assess the client's level of ability to assist with the bath. *Comments:*	☐	☐	☐	
2. Assess the client's level of comfort with the procedure. Check into potential cultural, sexual, or generational issues. *Comments:*	☐	☐	☐	
3. Assess the environment and equipment available. *Comments:*	☐	☐	☐	
Planning/Expected Outcomes				
1. Clients will be cleaned without damage to their skin. *Comments:*	☐	☐	☐	
2. Clients' privacy will be maintained throughout the procedure. *Comments:*	☐	☐	☐	
3. Clients will participate in own hygiene as much as possible. *Comments:*	☐	☐	☐	
4. Clients will not become overly tired or experience increased pain, cold, or discomfort as a result of the bath. *Comments:*	☐	☐	☐	
Implementation				
1. Check client's identification band and explain procedure before beginning. Assess client's preferences about bathing. *Comments:*	☐	☐	☐	
2. Prepare environment: close doors and windows, adjust temperature, provide time for elimination, and provide privacy. *Comments:*	☐	☐	☐	

continued on the following page

continued from the previous page

Procedure 29-19	Able to Perform	Able to Perform with Assistance	Unable to Perform	Initials and Date
3. Wash hands. Apply gloves. *Comments:*	☐	☐	☐	
4. Lower side rail on the side close to you. Position client in a comfortable position close to the side near you. *Comments:*	☐	☐	☐	
5. If bath blankets are available, place bath blanket over top sheet. Remove top sheet and client's gown. Bath blanket should be folded to expose only the area being cleaned at that time. *Comments:*	☐	☐	☐	
6. Fill washbasin two-thirds full. Permit client to test temperature of water with hand. Water should be changed when a soap film develops or water becomes soiled. *Comments:*	☐	☐	☐	
7. Wet the washcloth and wring it out. *Comments:*	☐	☐	☐	
8. Make a bath mitten with the washcloth. Some facilities use premoistened cloths when giving baths rather than a washcloth and washbasin. Use the cloths as a washcloth and proceed with the following steps. *Comments:*	☐	☐	☐	
9. Wash the client's face, neck, and ears. Shave the client if needed. *Comments:*	☐	☐	☐	
10. Wash the arms, forearms, hands, and axilla. Rinse and dry well. Apply deodorant or powder if desired. *Comments:*	☐	☐	☐	
11. Wash the chest and abdomen. Rinse and dry all skin areas well. Replace bath blanket over chest and abdomen. *Comments:*	☐	☐	☐	

Procedure 29-19	Able to Perform	Able to Perform with Assistance	Unable to Perform	Initials and Date
12. Wash the legs and feet. Gently wash the legs of clients with deep vein thrombosis (DVT) or other coagulation issues; do not use firm strokes. Rinse legs and dry well. Do not massage legs as an embolus may occur. *Comments:*	☐	☐	☐	
13. Wash the back. Assist the client into a prone or side-lying position facing away from you. Wash back and buttocks using long, firm strokes. Rinse and pat well. Give back rub and apply lotion. *Comments:*	☐	☐	☐	
14. Assist the client to a supine position. Perform perineal care. *Comments:*	☐	☐	☐	
15. Apply lotion and powder as desired. Apply clean gown. *Comments:*	☐	☐	☐	
16. Wash hands. *Comments:*	☐	☐	☐	
Evaluation				
1. Client was cleaned adequately without skin damage. *Comments:*	☐	☐	☐	
2. The client's modesty was maintained throughout the procedure. *Comments:*	☐	☐	☐	
3. The client participated in the procedure as much as possible. *Comments:*	☐	☐	☐	
4. The client remained comfortable during the procedure. *Comments:*	☐	☐	☐	

Checklist for Procedure 29-20   Perineal Care

Name _____   Date _____

School _____

Instructor _____

Course _____

Procedure 29-20 Perineal Care	Able to Perform	Able to Perform with Assistance	Unable to Perform	Initials and Date
Assessment				
1. Evaluate client status; level of consciousness, ability to ambulate, ability to perform self-care, frequency of urination and defecation, skin condition. *Comments:*	☐	☐	☐	
2. Identify cultural preferences for perineal care. *Comments:*	☐	☐	☐	
3. Assess the client's perineal health. Ask the male client if he has any perineal/genital itching or discomfort. Ask the female client if she has any urethral, vaginal, or anal discharge. *Comments:*	☐	☐	☐	
4. Determine if the client is incontinent of urine or stool. *Comments:*	☐	☐	☐	
5. Assess whether the client has recently had perineal/genital surgery. *Comments:*	☐	☐	☐	
Planning/Expected Outcomes				
1. Perineum and genitalia will be dry, clean, and free of secretions and unpleasant odor. *Comments:*	☐	☐	☐	
2. The client will report feeling comfortable and clean in perineal area. *Comments:*	☐	☐	☐	
3. The client will not experience discomfort or undue embarrassment during the procedure. *Comments:*	☐	☐	☐	

continued on the following page

continued from the previous page

Procedure 29-20	Able to Perform	Able to Perform with Assistance	Unable to Perform	Initials and Date
4. The perineum will be free of skin breakdown or irritation. *Comments:*	☐	☐	☐	
Implementation				
1. Check client's identification band and explain procedure before beginning. Wash hands and wear gloves. If appropriate and splashing is likely, wear gown, mask, and goggles. *Comments:*	☐	☐	☐	
2. Close privacy curtain or door. *Comments:*	☐	☐	☐	
3. Position client. *Comments:*	☐	☐	☐	
4. Place waterproof pads under the client in the bed or under bedpan if used. *Comments:*	☐	☐	☐	
5. Remove fecal debris with toilet paper and dispose in toilet. *Comments:*	☐	☐	☐	
6. Spray perineum with washing solution if indicated. *Comments:*	☐	☐	☐	
7. Wash perineum with wet washcloths (front to back on females). Wash the penis on the male. *Comments:*	☐	☐	☐	
8. Examine gluteal folds, scrotal folds, and vulva for debris. *Comments:*	☐	☐	☐	
9. If soap is used, spray area with clean water from the peri-bottle. *Comments:*	☐	☐	☐	
10. Change gloves. *Comments:*	☐	☐	☐	

Procedure 29-20	Able to Perform	Able to Perform with Assistance	Unable to Perform	Initials and Date
11. Dry perineum carefully with towel. *Comments:*	☐	☐	☐	
12. If indicated, apply barrier lotion or ointment. *Comments:*	☐	☐	☐	
13. Reposition or dress the client as appropriate. *Comments:*	☐	☐	☐	
14. Dispose of linens and garbage according to hospital policy. *Comments:*	☐	☐	☐	
15. Wash hands. *Comments:*	☐	☐	☐	
16. Deodorize room if appropriate. *Comments:*	☐	☐	☐	

Evaluation

	Able to Perform	Able to Perform with Assistance	Unable to Perform	Initials and Date
1. The perineum and genitalia are dry, clean, and free of secretions and unpleasant odors. *Comments:*	☐	☐	☐	
2. The client reports feeling comfortable and clean in the perineal area. *Comments:*	☐	☐	☐	
3. The client did not experience discomfort or undue embarrassment during the procedure. *Comments:*	☐	☐	☐	

Checklist for Procedure 29-21   Routine Catheter Care

Name _____ Date _____

School _____

Instructor _____

Course _____

Procedure 29-21 Routine Catheter Care	Able to Perform	Able to Perform with Assistance	Unable to Perform	Initials and Date
Assessment				
1. Assess catheter patency and urine color, consistency, and amount while doing the care. *Comments:*	☐	☐	☐	
2. Determine the condition of the urinary meatus and perineal area to monitor for redness, swelling, drainage, stool, or vaginal discharge, as indicators of infection. *Comments:*	☐	☐	☐	
3. Determine the client's emotional reaction and feelings related to the catheter. *Comments:*	☐	☐	☐	
Planning/Expected Outcomes				
1. The client will be free of signs and symptoms of urinary tract infection. *Comments:*	☐	☐	☐	
2. The client will understand the reason for the catheter and related care. *Comments:*	☐	☐	☐	
3. The meatus and surrounding area will be clean and free of drainage. *Comments:*	☐	☐	☐	
Implementation				
1. Check client's identification band and explain procedure before beginning. Wash hands. *Comments:*	☐	☐	☐	
2. Check institutional protocol or care plan. *Comments:*	☐	☐	☐	
3. Provide privacy. *Comments:*	☐	☐	☐	

continued on the following page

continued from the previous page

Procedure 29-21	Able to Perform	Able to Perform with Assistance	Unable to Perform	Initials and Date
4. Place client in supine position and expose perineal area and catheter. *Comments:*	☐	☐	☐	
5. Place waterproof pad under client. *Comments:*	☐	☐	☐	
6. Put on clean gloves. *Comments:*	☐	☐	☐	
7. After performing perineal care (Basic Procedure 29-20), cleanse meatus if there is excessive purulent drainage with nonirritating antiseptic solution on cotton balls. *Comments:*	☐	☐	☐	
8. Cleanse catheter from meatus out to end of catheter, taking care not to pull on catheter. *Comments:*	☐	☐	☐	
9. Be sure to repeat catheter care anytime it becomes soiled with stool or other drainage. *Comments:*	☐	☐	☐	
10. Place linen or cotton balls in proper receptacle for laundry or disposal. *Comments:*	☐	☐	☐	
11. Wash hands. *Comments:*	☐	☐	☐	
Evaluation				
1. The client is free of signs and symptoms of urinary tract infection. *Comments:*	☐	☐	☐	
2. The client understands the reason for the catheter and related care. *Comments:*	☐	☐	☐	
3. The meatus and surrounding area are clean, intact, and free of drainage. *Comments:*	☐	☐	☐	

Checklist for Procedure 29-22   Oral Care

Name _____ Date _____

School _____

Instructor _____

Course _____

Procedure 29-22 Oral Care	Able to Perform	Able to Perform with Assistance	Unable to Perform	Initials and Date
Assessment				
1. Assess whether the client is able to assist with oral care and to what extent. *Comments:*	☐	☐	☐	
2. Evaluate whether the client has an understanding of proper oral hygiene. *Comments:*	☐	☐	☐	
3. Check whether the client has dentures. *Comments:*	☐	☐	☐	
4. Assess the condition of the client's mouth. *Comments:*	☐	☐	☐	
5. Assess whether inflammation, bleeding, infection, or ulceration is present. *Comments:*	☐	☐	☐	
6. Assess what cultural practices to consider. *Comments:*	☐	☐	☐	
7. Assess whether there are any appliances or devices present in the client's mouth, such as braces, endotracheal tube, or bridgework. *Comments:*	☐	☐	☐	
8. Check that the proper equipment is available to perform oral care. *Comments:*	☐	☐	☐	
Planning/Expected Outcomes				
1. Client's mouth, teeth, gums, and lips will be clean and free of food particles. *Comments:*	☐	☐	☐	

continued on the following page

continued from the previous page

Procedure 29-22	Able to Perform	Able to Perform with Assistance	Unable to Perform	Initials and Date
2. Any inflammation, bleeding, infection, or ulceration present will be noted and treated. *Comments:*	☐	☐	☐	
3. The oral mucosa will be clean, intact, and well hydrated. *Comments:*	☐	☐	☐	

Implementation

Self-Care Client: Flossing and Brushing

	Able to Perform	Able to Perform with Assistance	Unable to Perform	Initials and Date
1. Check client's identification band and explain procedure before beginning. Assemble articles for flossing and brushing. *Comments:*	☐	☐	☐	
2. Provide privacy. *Comments:*	☐	☐	☐	
3. Place the client in a high-Fowler's position. *Comments:*	☐	☐	☐	
4. Wash hands and apply gloves. *Comments:*	☐	☐	☐	
5. Arrange articles within the client's reach. *Comments:*	☐	☐	☐	
6. Assist client with flossing and brushing as necessary. Position mirror, emesis basin, and water with straw near the client and a towel across the client's chest. *Comments:*	☐	☐	☐	
7. Assist the client with rinsing mouth. *Comments:*	☐	☐	☐	
8. Reposition client, raise side rails, and place call button within reach. *Comments:*	☐	☐	☐	
9. Rinse, dry, and return articles to proper place. *Comments:*	☐	☐	☐	
10. Remove gloves, cleanse hands, and document care. *Comments:*	☐	☐	☐	

Procedure 29-22	Able to Perform	Able to Perform with Assistance	Unable to Perform	Initials and Date
Self-Care Client: Denture Care				
11. Assemble articles for denture cleaning. *Comments:*	☐	☐	☐	
12. Provide privacy. *Comments:*	☐	☐	☐	
13. Assist client to a high-Fowler's position. *Comments:*	☐	☐	☐	
14. Wash hands and apply gloves. *Comments:*	☐	☐	☐	
15. Assist the client with denture removal. Place in denture cup. *Comments:*	☐	☐	☐	
16. Apply toothpaste to brush and brush dentures either with cool water in the emesis basin or under running water in the sink. Pad sink with towel to protect dentures in case they are dropped. *Comments:*	☐	☐	☐	
17. Rinse thoroughly. *Comments:*	☐	☐	☐	
18. Assist client with rinsing mouth and replacing dentures. *Comments:*	☐	☐	☐	
19. Reposition the client, raise side rails, and place call button within reach. *Comments:*	☐	☐	☐	
20. Rinse, dry, and return articles to proper place. *Comments:*	☐	☐	☐	
21. Remove gloves, and wash hands. *Comments:*	☐	☐	☐	

continued on the following page

continued from the previous page

Procedure 29-22	Able to Perform	Able to Perform with Assistance	Unable to Perform	Initials and Date
Full-Care Client: Brushing and Flossing				
22. Assemble articles for flossing and brushing. *Comments:*	☐	☐	☐	
23. Provide privacy. *Comments:*	☐	☐	☐	
24. Wash hands and apply gloves. *Comments:*	☐	☐	☐	
25. Position the client as condition allows: high Fowler's, semi-Fowler's, or lateral position, head turned toward side. *Comments:*	☐	☐	☐	
26. Place towel across the client's chest or under face and mouth, if head is turned to one side. *Comments:*	☐	☐	☐	
27. Moisten toothbrush or toothette, apply small amount of toothpaste, and brush teeth and gums. *Comments:*	☐	☐	☐	
28. Floss between all teeth. *Comments:*	☐	☐	☐	
29. Assist the client in rinsing mouth. *Comments:*	☐	☐	☐	
30. Reapply toothpaste and brush the teeth and gums. *Comments:*	☐	☐	☐	
31. Assist the client in rinsing and drying mouth. *Comments:*	☐	☐	☐	
32. Apply lip moisturizer, if appropriate. *Comments:*	☐	☐	☐	
33. Reposition the client, raise side rails, and place call button within reach. *Comments:*	☐	☐	☐	

Procedure 29-22	Able to Perform	Able to Perform with Assistance	Unable to Perform	Initials and Date
34. Rinse, dry, and return articles to proper place. *Comments:*	☐	☐	☐	
35. Remove gloves and wash hands. *Comments:*	☐	☐	☐	
Clients at Risk for or with an Alteration of the Oral Cavity				
36. Follow Actions 22–24. *Comments:*	☐	☐	☐	

37. Bleeding:
  a. Assess oral cavity for signs of bleeding.
  b. Proceed with the actions for oral care for a full-care client, except:
    • Do not floss.
    • Use a soft toothbrush, toothette, or a tongue blade padded with 3×3 gauze sponges to swab teeth and gums.
    • Dispose of padded tongue blade into a biohazard bag according to institutional policy.
    • Rinse with tepid water.
Comments:
	☐	☐	☐	

38. Infection or ulceration:
  a. Assess oral cavity for signs of infection.
  b. Culture lesions as ordered.
  c. Proceed with the actions for oral care for a full-care client except:
    • Do not floss.
    • Use prescribed antiseptic solution.
    • Use a tongue blade padded with 3×3 gauze sponges to gently swab the teeth and gums.
    • Dispose of padded tongue blade into a biohazard bag according to institutional policy.
    • Rinse mouth with tepid water.
    • Apply additional solution as prescribed.
Comments:
	☐	☐	☐	

Unconscious (Comatose) Client:				
39. Follow Actions 22–24. *Comments:*	☐	☐	☐	
40. Place the client in a lateral position, with head turned toward the side. *Comments:*	☐	☐	☐	

continued on the following page

continued from the previous page

Procedure 29-22	Able to Perform	Able to Perform with Assistance	Unable to Perform	Initials and Date
41. Use a floss holder and floss between all teeth. *Comments:*	☐	☐	☐	
42. Moisten toothbrush or toothette, and brush the teeth and gums using friction in a circular motion. Do not use toothpaste. *Comments:*	☐	☐	☐	
43. After flossing and brushing, rinse mouth with an Asepto syringe (do not force water into the mouth) and perform oral suction. *Comments:*	☐	☐	☐	
44. Dry the client's mouth. *Comments:*	☐	☐	☐	
45. Apply lip moisturizer. *Comments:*	☐	☐	☐	
46. Leave the client in a lateral position with head turned toward side for 30–60 minutes after oral care. Suction one more time. Remove the towel from under the client's mouth and face. *Comments:*	☐	☐	☐	
47. Dispose of any contaminated items in a biohazard bag and clean, dry, and return all articles to appropriate place. *Comments:*	☐	☐	☐	
48. Remove gloves and wash hands. *Comments:*	☐	☐	☐	
Evaluation				
1. The client's mouth, teeth, gums, and lips are clean and free of food particles. *Comments:*	☐	☐	☐	
2. Inflammation, bleeding, infection, or ulceration are noted and cared for. *Comments:*	☐	☐	☐	

Procedure 29-22	Able to Perform	Able to Perform with Assistance	Unable to Perform	Initials and Date
3. The oral mucosa is clean, intact, and well hydrated. *Comments:*	☐	☐	☐	
4. The oral care was performed with a minimum of trauma to the client. *Comments:*	☐	☐	☐	

Checklist for Procedure 29-23   Eye Care

Name _____   Date _____

School _____

Instructor _____

Course _____

Procedure 29-23 Eye Care	Able to Perform	Able to Perform with Assistance	Unable to Perform	Initials and Date
Assessment				
1. Determine if the client is wearing contact lenses or has an ocular prosthesis. *Comments:*	☐	☐	☐	
2. Determine availability of eye care supplies. If the client can tell you what kind of eye care products he or she normally uses, ask for these products or have a family member bring them from home. *Comments:*	☐	☐	☐	
3. Assess whether the client can do his or her own eye care. If not, evaluate what kind of assistance the client needs. *Comments:*	☐	☐	☐	
Planning/Expected Outcomes				
1. The client's contact lenses will be safely removed and stored. *Comments:*	☐	☐	☐	
2. The client's ocular prosthesis will be safely removed, cleaned, and either stored or returned to the client's eye socket. *Comments:*	☐	☐	☐	
3. The client's contacts or prosthesis will be cared for with a minimum of trauma to the client's eyes. *Comments:*	☐	☐	☐	
4. The client's eyes will be free of crusts and exudate. *Comments:*	☐	☐	☐	
Implementation				
Artificial Eye Removal 1. Check client's identification band and explain procedure before beginning. Inquire about client's care regimen and gather equipment accordingly. *Comments:*	☐	☐	☐	

continued on the following page

continued from the previous page

Procedure 29-23	Able to Perform	Able to Perform with Assistance	Unable to Perform	Initials and Date
2. Provide privacy. *Comments:*	☐	☐	☐	
3. Wash hands; apply gloves. *Comments:*	☐	☐	☐	
4. Place client in a semi-Fowler's position. *Comments:*	☐	☐	☐	
5. Place the cotton balls in an emesis basin filled halfway with warm water. *Comments:*	☐	☐	☐	
6. Place 3 × 3 gauze sponges in bottom of second emesis basin and fill halfway with mild soap and tepid water. *Comments:*	☐	☐	☐	
7. Grasp and squeeze excess water from a cotton ball. Cleanse the eyelid with the moistened cotton ball, starting at the inner canthus and moving outward toward the outer canthus. After each use, dispose of cotton ball in biohazard bag. Repeat procedure until eyelid is clean (without dried secretions). *Comments:*	☐	☐	☐	

8. Remove the artificial eye:
  a. Using dominant hand, raise the client's upper eyelid with index finger and depress the lower eyelid with thumb.
  b. Cup nondominant hand under the client's lower eyelid.
  c. Apply slight pressure with index finger between the brow and the artificial eye and remove it. Place it in an emesis basin filled with warm, soapy water.
Comments:
	☐	☐	☐	

9. Grasp a moistened cotton ball and cleanse around the edge of the eye socket. Dispose of the soiled cotton ball into biohazard bag. *Comments:*	☐	☐	☐	
10. Inspect the eye socket for irritation, drainage, or crusting. *Comments:*	☐	☐	☐	

Procedure 29-23	Able to Perform	Able to Perform with Assistance	Unable to Perform	Initials and Date

11. If irrigation is ordered:
   a. Lower the head of the bed and place the client in a supine position. Place protector pan on bed; turn head toward socket side and slightly extend neck.
   b. Fill the irrigation syringe with the prescribed amount and type of irrigating solution.
   c. With nondominant hand, separate the eyelids with your forefinger and thumb while resting fingers on the brow and cheekbone.
   d. Hold the irrigating syringe in dominant hand, several inches above the inner canthus; with thumb, gently apply pressure on the plunger, directing the flow of solution from the inner canthus along the conjunctival sac.
   e. Irrigate until the prescribed amount of solution has been used.
   f. Wipe the eyelids with a moistened cotton ball after irrigating. Dispose of the soiled cotton ball into biohazard bag.
   g. Pat the skin dry with the towel.
   h. Return the client to a semi-Fowler's position.
   i. Remove gloves, wash hands, and apply clean gloves.
Comments:
	☐	☐	☐	

12. Rub the artificial eye between index finger and thumb in the basin of warm, soapy water. *Comments:*	☐	☐	☐	
13. Rinse the prosthesis under running water or place in the clean basin of tepid water. Do not dry the prosthesis. *Comments:*	☐	☐	☐	

14. Reinsert the prosthesis:
   a. With the thumb of the nondominant hand, raise and hold the upper eyelid open.
   b. With the dominant hand, grasp the artificial eye so that the indented part is facing the client's nose and slide it under the upper eyelid as far as possible.
   c. Depress the lower lid.
   d. Pull the lower lid forward to cover the edge of the prosthesis.
Comments:
	☐	☐	☐	

15. Place the cleaned artificial eye in a labeled container with saline or tap water. *Comments:*	☐	☐	☐	

continued on the following page

continued from the previous page

Procedure 29-23	Able to Perform	Able to Perform with Assistance	Unable to Perform	Initials and Date
16. Grasp a moistened cotton ball and squeeze out excessive moisture. Wipe the eyelid from the inner to the outer canthus. Dispose of the soiled cotton ball into biohazard bag. *Comments:*	☐	☐	☐	
17. Clean, dry, and replace equipment. *Comments:*	☐	☐	☐	
18. Reposition the client, raise side rails, and place call light within reach. *Comments:*	☐	☐	☐	
19. Dispose of biohazard bag according to institutional policy. *Comments:*	☐	☐	☐	
20. Remove gloves and wash hands. *Comments:*	☐	☐	☐	
Contact Lens Removal				
21. Assess level of assistance needed and provide privacy. *Comments:*	☐	☐	☐	
22. Wash hands. *Comments:*	☐	☐	☐	
23. Assist the client to a semi-Fowler's position if needed. *Comments:*	☐	☐	☐	
24. Drape a clean towel over the client's chest. *Comments:*	☐	☐	☐	
25. Prepare the lens storage case with the prescribed solution. *Comments:*	☐	☐	☐	
26. Instruct the client to look straight ahead. Assess the location of the lens. If it is not on the cornea, either you or the client should gently move the lens toward the cornea with pad of index finger. *Comments:*	☐	☐	☐	

Procedure 29-23	Able to Perform	Able to Perform with Assistance	Unable to Perform	Initials and Date
27. Remove the lens. a. Hard lens: • Cup nondominant hand under the eye. • Gently place index finger on the outside corner of the eye, pull toward the temple, and ask the client to blink. Catch the lens in your nondominant hand. b. Soft lens: • With nondominant hand, separate the eyelid with your thumb and middle finger. • With the index finger of the dominant hand gently placed on the lower edge of the lens, slide the lens downward onto the sclera and gently squeeze the lens. • Release the top eyelid (continue holding the lower lid down) and remove the lens with your index finger and thumb. • If lens cannot be extracted using fingers, secure a suction cup to remove the contact lens. *Comments:*	☐	☐	☐	
28. Store the lens in the correct compartment of the case. Label with the client's name. *Comments:*	☐	☐	☐	
29. Repeat Actions 27 and 28 for the second lens. *Comments:*	☐	☐	☐	
30. Assess eyes for irritation or redness. *Comments:*	☐	☐	☐	
31. Store the lens case in a safe place. *Comments:*	☐	☐	☐	
32. Dispose of soiled articles and clean and return reusable articles to proper location. *Comments:*	☐	☐	☐	
33. Reposition the client, raise side rails, and place call light within reach. *Comments:*	☐	☐	☐	
34. Remove gloves and wash hands. *Comments:*	☐	☐	☐	

continued from the previous page

Procedure 29-23	Able to Perform	Able to Perform with Assistance	Unable to Perform	Initials and Date
Evaluation				
1. Client's contact lenses were safely removed and stored. *Comments:*	☐	☐	☐	
2. Client's ocular prosthesis was safely removed, cleaned, and either stored or returned to the client's eye socket. *Comments:*	☐	☐	☐	
3. Client's contacts or prosthesis were cared for with a minimum of trauma to the client's eyes. *Comments:*	☐	☐	☐	
4. Client's eyes are free of crusts and exudates. *Comments:*	☐	☐	☐	
5. Client is comfortable. *Comments:*	☐	☐	☐	

Checklist for Procedure 29-24 Giving a Back Rub

Name _____ Date _____

School _____

Instructor _____

Course _____

Procedure 29-24 Giving a Back Rub	Able to Perform	Able to Perform with Assistance	Unable to Perform	Initials and Date
Assessment				
1. Assess the client's willingness to have a massage. *Comments:*	☐	☐	☐	
2. Assess the client for contraindications of a back rub. Conditions include open sores or lesions, vertebral fractures, burns, or signs of decubitus ulcers. *Comments:*	☐	☐	☐	
3. Assess any limitations the client has in positioning. *Comments:*	☐	☐	☐	
4. Assess the client for fatigue, stiffness, or soreness in the back and shoulders. *Comments:*	☐	☐	☐	
5. Assess the client for anxiety or emotional disturbances. *Comments:*	☐	☐	☐	
6. If possible, have the client quantify the degree of discomfort using a 1 to 10 rating scale. *Comments:*	☐	☐	☐	
Planning/Expected Outcomes				
1. The client will experience a reduction in tension, anxiety, pain, and fatigue. *Comments:*	☐	☐	☐	
2. The client's circulation to the back is improved. *Comments:*	☐	☐	☐	
3. The nurse will establish a better rapport with the client. *Comments:*	☐	☐	☐	

continued on the following page

continued from the previous page

Procedure 29-24	Able to Perform	Able to Perform with Assistance	Unable to Perform	Initials and Date
Implementation				
1. Check client's identification band and explain procedure before beginning. Wash your hands and apply gloves if necessary. *Comments:*	☐	☐	☐	
2. Help client to a prone or side-lying position. *Comments:*	☐	☐	☐	
3. Drape the bath blanket, and undo the client's gown, exposing the back, shoulder, and sacral area, but keeping the remainder of the body covered. *Comments:*	☐	☐	☐	
4. Pour a small amount of lotion in your hand and warm between your palms for a few moments. Baby powder may be substituted for oils or lotions. *Comments:*	☐	☐	☐	
5. Begin in the sacral area with smooth, circular strokes, moving upward toward the shoulders. Gradually lengthen the strokes to the upper back, scapula, and upper arms. Apply firm, continuous pressure without breaking contact with the client. *Comments:*	☐	☐	☐	
6. Assess client's back as you are massaging for areas of redness and signs of decreased circulation. *Comments:*	☐	☐	☐	
7. Provide a firm, kneading massage to areas of increased tension, such as the shoulders and gluteal muscles, if desired. *Comments:*	☐	☐	☐	
8. Complete the massage with long, very light brush strokes, using the tips of the fingers. *Comments:*	☐	☐	☐	
9. Wipe off excess lubricant and cover the client. *Comments:*	☐	☐	☐	
10. Wash hands. *Comments:*	☐	☐	☐	

Procedure 29-24	Able to Perform	Able to Perform with Assistance	Unable to Perform	Initials and Date
Evaluation				
1. Client experienced a reduction in tension, anxiety, pain, and fatigue. *Comments:*	☐	☐	☐	
2. Nurse established better rapport with the client. *Comments:*	☐	☐	☐	

Checklist for Procedure 29-25   Shaving a Client

Name _____   Date _____

School _____

Instructor _____

Course _____

Procedure 29-25 **Shaving a Client**	Able to **Perform**	**Able to Perform with Assistance**	**Unable to Perform**	**Initials and Date**
Assessment				
1. Assess whether the client is able to perform self-care. *Comments:*	☐	☐	☐	
2. Assess the client's skin for areas of redness, skin breakdown, moles, or skin lesions. *Comments:*	☐	☐	☐	
3. Assess whether the client has a bleeding tendency or is on anticoagulatnts. If there is an increased risk of bleeding, an electric razor is used. *Comments:*	☐	☐	☐	
4. Assess the client's ability to manipulate the razor. *Comments:*	☐	☐	☐	
5. Assess the client's preference for the type of shaving, type of equipment, and type of lotion. *Comments:*	☐	☐	☐	
Planning/Expected Outcomes				
1. The client will be neat and well-groomed. *Comments:*	☐	☐	☐	
2. The client's skin integrity will remain intact. *Comments:*	☐	☐	☐	
3. The client will attain a sense of independence. *Comments:*	☐	☐	☐	
4. The client will be comfortable after the procedure. *Comments:*	☐	☐	☐	

continued on the following page

continued from the previous page

Procedure 29-25	Able to Perform	Able to Perform with Assistance	Unable to Perform	Initials and Date
Implementation				
1. Check client's identification band and explain procedure before beginning. Wash hands and apply gloves. *Comments:*	☐	☐	☐	
2. If the client can shave himself, set up the equipment and supplies, and watch the client for safety. Adjust lighting as needed. *Comments:*	☐	☐	☐	
3. Place a towel over the client's chest and shoulder. *Comments:*	☐	☐	☐	
4. Raise the bed to a comfortable height. *Comments:*	☐	☐	☐	
5. Fill a washbasin with warm water. Check temperature for comfort. *Comments:*	☐	☐	☐	
6. Place the washcloth in the basin and wring out thoroughly. Apply cloth over the client's face. Remove washcloth. *Comments:*	☐	☐	☐	
7. Apply shaving cream. *Comments:*	☐	☐	☐	
8. Take the razor in the dominant hand and hold it at a 45-degree angle to the client's skin. Start shaving across one side of the client's face. Use the nondominant hand to gently pull the skin taut while shaving. Use short, firm strokes in the direction hair grows. Use short, downward strokes over the upper lip area. *Comments:*	☐	☐	☐	
9. Rinse the razor in water as cream accumulates. *Comments:*	☐	☐	☐	
10. Check the face to see if all the facial hair is removed. *Comments:*	☐	☐	☐	

Procedure 29-25	Able to Perform	Able to Perform with Assistance	Unable to Perform	Initials and Date
11. Rinse the face thoroughly with a moistened washcloth. *Comments:*	☐	☐	☐	
12. Dry the face thoroughly and apply aftershave lotion if desired. *Comments:*	☐	☐	☐	
13. Assist the client to inspect the results of the shave. *Comments:*	☐	☐	☐	
14. Dispose of equipment in proper receptacle. *Comments:*	☐	☐	☐	
15. Wash hands. *Comments:*	☐	☐	☐	
Evaluation				
1. Client is neat and well-groomed. *Comments:*	☐	☐	☐	
2. Client's skin integrity remained intact. *Comments:*	☐	☐	☐	
3. If the client was able to shave or able to assist, the client attained a sense of independence. *Comments:*	☐	☐	☐	
4. Client is comfortable following the procedure. *Comments:*	☐	☐	☐	

Checklist for Procedure 29-26   Applying Antiembolic Stockings

Name _____ Date _____

School _____

Instructor _____

Course _____

Procedure 29-26 Applying Antiembolic Stockings	Able to Perform	Able to Perform with Assistance	Unable to Perform	Initials and Date
Assessment				
1. Assess the condition of the client's lower extremities, noting edema, color, temperature, intact skin, ulcers, or infections. *Comments:*	☐	☐	☐	
2. Assess the quality and equality of peripheral pulses in the legs (either dorsalis pedis or posterior tibial pulses) to determine circulatory status. *Comments:*	☐	☐	☐	
3. Assess the client's understanding of the reasons for, and the use of, the antiembolic stockings to determine the amount of client teaching required. *Comments:*	☐	☐	☐	
4. Assess the client for signs and symptoms of deep vein thrombosis, such as increased calf size or color change. *Comments:*	☐	☐	☐	
Planning/Expected Outcomes				
1. The client will experience no signs or symptoms of deep venous thrombosis or thrombophlebitis. *Comments:*	☐	☐	☐	
2. The client's venous return will be improved. *Comments:*	☐	☐	☐	
3. The client's popliteal, posterior tibial, and dorsalis pedis pulses will remain intact while stockings are in place. *Comments:*	☐	☐	☐	
4. The client will have good circulation while stockings are in place. *Comments:*	☐	☐	☐	

continued on the following page

continued from the previous page

Procedure 29-26	Able to Perform	Able to Perform with Assistance	Unable to Perform	Initials and Date
Implementation				
1. Check client's identification band and explain procedure before beginning. Wash hands. *Comments:*	☐	☐	☐	
2. Review the orders with the client, including the reason for the stockings and the type of stockings ordered, for example, knee- or thigh-high. *Comments:*	☐	☐	☐	
3. With the client in supine position in bed, measure the client's leg for the correct size: Thigh-high stockings: from Achilles tendon to the gluteal fold, circumference of the midthigh; Below-the-knee stockings: from the Achilles tendon to the popliteal fold, circumference of the midcalf. *Comments:*	☐	☐	☐	
4. Compare the obtained measurements with the package to ascertain proper size. *Comments:*	☐	☐	☐	
5. Apply stockings. Keep client in supine position until stockings are applied. *Comments:*	☐	☐	☐	
6. Open the package and turn a stocking inside out over hand and arm. Place hand deep enough inside the stocking to grasp the stocking toe. *Comments:*	☐	☐	☐	
7. Using the hand inside the stocking, hold onto the client's toe. Invert the stocking with the other hand and pull it over the hand and the client's toes. Release toes. *Comments:*	☐	☐	☐	
8. Hold each side of the stocking and pull it from the client's toes to the heel in one motion. *Comments:*	☐	☐	☐	
9. Continuing to hold each side of the stocking, firmly pull the stocking up by using the thumbs to guide the stocking upward over the ankles and up the client's leg. *Comments:*	☐	☐	☐	

Procedure 29-26	Able to Perform	Able to Perform with Assistance	Unable to Perform	Initials and Date
10. Repeat with the other leg if necessary. *Comments:*	☐	☐	☐	
11. Smooth and remove any wrinkles in the stockings. *Comments:*	☐	☐	☐	
12. Assess circulatory and neurostatus of feet (CMS: circulatory, movement, sensation). *Comments:*	☐	☐	☐	
13. Wash hands. *Comments:*	☐	☐	☐	
Evaluation				
1. The client has not experienced any signs or symptoms of deep venous thrombosis or thrombophlebitis. *Comments:*	☐	☐	☐	
2. Client's venous return is improved. *Comments:*	☐	☐	☐	
3. The client's popliteal, posterior tibial, and dorsalis pedis pulses remain intact while stockings are in place. *Comments:*	☐	☐	☐	
4. The client has good circulation while stockings are in place, as evidenced by warm skin temperature, capillary return within normal limits, sensation within normal limits, and no edema in either extremities. *Comments:*	☐	☐	☐	

Checklist for Procedure 29-27   Assisting with a Bedpan or Urinal

Name _____ Date _____

School _____

Instructor _____

Course _____

Procedure 29-27 **Assisting with a Bedpan or Urinal**	Able to Perform	Able to Perform with Assistance	Unable to Perform	Initials and Date
Assessment				
1. Assess your equipment. *Comments:*	☐	☐	☐	
2. Assess how much the client can assist in positioning and removing the bedpan. *Comments:*	☐	☐	☐	
3. Check whether the client is confused, combative, in traction, or immobile. *Comments:*	☐	☐	☐	
4. Check for casts, braces, or dressings that need protecting from accidental contamination with waste products. *Comments:*	☐	☐	☐	
5. Check for privacy and unexpected interruptions. *Comments:*	☐	☐	☐	
6. Assess if the client has orders to record intake and output. *Comments:*	☐	☐	☐	
Planning/Expected Outcomes				
1. Client will be able to void and defecate when necessary. *Comments:*	☐	☐	☐	
2. Client will have as much privacy and comfort as allowable, given physical condition. *Comments:*	☐	☐	☐	
3. Intake and output will be accurately measured as needed. *Comments:*	☐	☐	☐	

continued on the following page

continued from the previous page

Procedure 29-27	Able to Perform	Able to Perform with Assistance	Unable to Perform	Initials and Date
4. The urinal or bedpan will be placed without skin damage. *Comments:*	☐	☐	☐	
5. The bedpan will be removed and emptied without spillage. *Comments:*	☐	☐	☐	

Implementation

Positioning a Bedpan

	Able to Perform	Able to Perform with Assistance	Unable to Perform	Initials and Date
1. Check client's identification band and explain procedure before beginning. Close curtain or door. *Comments:*	☐	☐	☐	
2. Wash hands and apply gloves. *Comments:*	☐	☐	☐	
3. Lower head of bed so client is in supine position. *Comments:*	☐	☐	☐	
4. Elevate bed. *Comments:*	☐	☐	☐	
5. Assist client to side-lying position using side rail for support. *Comments:*	☐	☐	☐	
6. Powder edge of bedpan if necessary. *Comments:*	☐	☐	☐	
7. While holding the bedpan with one hand, help the client roll onto his or her back, while pushing against the bedpan (toward the center of the bed) to hold it in place. *Comments:*	☐	☐	☐	
8. Alternate: Help the client raise the hips using the overhead trapeze, and slide the pan in place. Alternate: If the client is unable to turn or raise hips, use a fracture pan instead of a bedpan. With a fracture pan, the flat side is placed toward the client's head. *Comments:*	☐	☐	☐	
9. Check placement of bedpan. *Comments:*	☐	☐	☐	

Procedure 29-27	Able to Perform	Able to Perform with Assistance	Unable to Perform	Initials and Date
10. If indicated, elevate head of bed to 45-degree angle or higher for comfort. Comments:	☐	☐	☐	
11. Place call light within reach; place side rails in upright position, lower bed, and provide privacy. Comments:	☐	☐	☐	
12. Remove gloves and wash hands. Comments:	☐	☐	☐	
Positioning a Urinal				
13. Repeat actions 1 and 2. Comments:	☐	☐	☐	
14. Lift the covers and place the urinal so the client may grasp the handle and position it. If the client cannot do this, you must position the urinal and place the penis into the opening. Comments:	☐	☐	☐	
15. Remove gloves and wash hands. Comments:	☐	☐	☐	
Removing a Bedpan				
16. Wash hands and apply gloves. Comments:	☐	☐	☐	
17. Gather toilet paper and washing supplies. Comments:	☐	☐	☐	
18. Lower head of bed to supine position. Comments:	☐	☐	☐	
19. While holding bedpan with one hand, roll client to side and remove the pan, being careful not to pull or shear skin sticking to the pan and being careful not to spill contents. Comments:	☐	☐	☐	

continued on the following page

continued from the previous page

Procedure 29-27	Able to Perform	Able to Perform with Assistance	Unable to Perform	Initials and Date
20. Assist with cleaning or wiping; always wipe from front to back. *Comments:*	☐	☐	☐	
21. Empty bedpan (observe and measure urine output and check for occult blood if ordered), clean bedpan, and store in proper place. *Comments:*	☐	☐	☐	
22. Remove soiled gloves. Wash hands. *Comments:*	☐	☐	☐	
23. Allow client to wash hands. *Comments:*	☐	☐	☐	
24. Place call light in reach; raise side rails. *Comments:*	☐	☐	☐	
25. Wash hands. *Comments:*	☐	☐	☐	
Removing a Urinal				
26. Wash hands and apply gloves. *Comments:*	☐	☐	☐	
27. Empty the urinal, measuring urine output if ordered, rinse the urinal, and replace it within the client's reach. Observe odor and color of urine before discarding. *Comments:*	☐	☐	☐	
28. Remove soiled gloves. Wash hands. *Comments:*	☐	☐	☐	
29. Allow client to wash hands. *Comments:*	☐	☐	☐	
30. Place call light within reach; raise side rails. *Comments:*	☐	☐	☐	

Procedure 29-27	Able to Perform	Able to Perform with Assistance	Unable to Perform	Initials and Date
31. Wash hands. *Comments:*	☐	☐	☐	

Evaluation

	Able to Perform	Able to Perform with Assistance	Unable to Perform	Initials and Date
1. The client was able to void or defecate as needed. *Comments:*	☐	☐	☐	
2. The client's request for assistance was answered promptly. *Comments:*	☐	☐	☐	
3. The bedpan or urinal was removed and emptied without spillage. *Comments:*	☐	☐	☐	
4. Ordered tests were performed, and samples were collected. *Comments:*	☐	☐	☐	
5. The client's skin integrity was maintained without skin shear or tearing. *Comments:*	☐	☐	☐	
6. The client was provided with as much privacy and comfort as possible. *Comments:*	☐	☐	☐	

Checklist for Procedure 29-28   Applying a Condom Catheter

Name _____   Date _____

School _____

Instructor _____

Course _____

Procedure 29-28 Applying a Condom Catheter	Able to Perform	Able to Perform with Assistance	Unable to Perform	Initials and Date
Assessment				
1. Assess skin integrity around the penis and perineal area. Comments:	☐	☐	☐	
2. Assess the client for ability to cooperate with the application and retention of the condom catheter to determine what type of teaching is necessary. Comments:	☐	☐	☐	
3. Assess the amount and pattern of urinary incontinence. Comments:	☐	☐	☐	
4. Assess for latex allergy. Comments:	☐	☐	☐	
Planning/Expected Outcomes				
1. The client will have a condom catheter in place without leakage or discomfort. Comments:	☐	☐	☐	
2. The client will have no skin irritation from the condom catheter. Comments:	☐	☐	☐	
3. The client will understand and cooperate with placement and retention of the condom catheter. Comments:	☐	☐	☐	
Implementation				
1. Check client's identification band and explain procedure before beginning. Wash hands. Comments:	☐	☐	☐	

continued on the following page

continued from the previous page

Procedure 29-28	Able to Perform	Able to Perform with Assistance	Unable to Perform	Initials and Date
2. Protect the client's privacy by closing the door and pulling curtains around the bed. *Comments:*	☐	☐	☐	
3. Position the client in a comfortable position. Raise the bed to a comfortable height for the nurse. *Comments:*	☐	☐	☐	
4. Apply non-sterile latex-free gloves. *Comments:*	☐	☐	☐	
5. Fold the client's gown across the abdomen and the sheet just below the pubic area. *Comments:*	☐	☐	☐	
6. Assess the client's penis for any signs of redness, irritation, or skin breakdown. *Comments:*	☐	☐	☐	
7. Clean the client's penis with warm, soapy water. Retract the foreskin on the uncircumcised male and clean thoroughly in folds. *Comments:*	☐	☐	☐	
8. Return the client's foreskin to its normal position. *Comments:*	☐	☐	☐	
9. Shave any excess hair around the base of the penis if required by institutional policy. *Comments:*	☐	☐	☐	
10. Rinse and dry the area. *Comments:*	☐	☐	☐	
11. If a condom kit is used, open the package containing the skin preparation. Wipe and apply skin preparation solution to the shaft of the penis. If the client has an erection, wait for termination of erection before applying the catheter. *Comments:*	☐	☐	☐	

Procedure 29-28	Able to Perform	Able to Perform with Assistance	Unable to Perform	Initials and Date
12. Apply the double-sided adhesive strip around the base of the client's penis in a spiral fashion. The strip is applied 1 inch from the proximal end of the penis. Do not completely encircle the penis or tightly encompass the penis. *Comments:*	☐	☐	☐	
13. Position the rolled condom at the distal portion of the penis and unroll it, covering the penis and the double-sided strip of adhesive. Leave a 1- to 2-inch space between the tip of the penis and the end of the condom. *Comments:*	☐	☐	☐	
14. Gently press the condom to the adhesive strip. *Comments:*	☐	☐	☐	
15. Attach the drainage bag tubing to the catheter tubing. Make sure the tubing lays over the client's legs, not under them. Secure the drainage bag to the side of the bed below the level of the client's bladder or to the drainage bag attached to the leg. *Comments:*	☐	☐	☐	
16. Determine that the condom and tubing are not twisted. *Comments:*	☐	☐	☐	
17. Cover the client. *Comments:*	☐	☐	☐	
18. Dispose of the used equipment in the appropriate receptacle. *Comments:*	☐	☐	☐	
19. Empty the bag, measure the client's urinary output, and record every 4 hours. Remove gloves and wash hands after procedure. *Comments:*	☐	☐	☐	
20. Return the client's bed to the lowest position and reposition client to comfortable or appropriate position. *Comments:*	☐	☐	☐	

continued from the previous page

Procedure 29-28	Able to Perform	Able to Perform with Assistance	Unable to Perform	Initials and Date
21. Remove the condom once a day to clean the area and assess the skin for signs of impaired skin integrity. *Comments:*	☐	☐	☐	
Evaluation				
1. The client's condom catheter is in place without leakage or discomfort. *Comments:*	☐	☐	☐	
2. The client does not have any skin irritation from the condom catheter. *Comments:*	☐	☐	☐	
3. The client understands the reason for, and cooperates with, the placement and retention of the condom catheter. *Comments:*	☐	☐	☐	

Checklist for Procedure 29-29   Administering an Enema

Name _____   Date _____

School _____

Instructor _____

Course _____

Procedure 29-29 **Administering an Enema**	Able to Perform	Able to Perform with Assistance	Unable to Perform	Initials and Date
Assessment				
1. Identify the type of enema and rationale of the ordered enema. *Comments:*	☐	☐	☐	
2. Assess the physical condition of the client. Determine if the client has bowel sounds. Assess for a history of constipation, hemorrhoids, or diverticulitis. Determine if the client is able to hold a side-lying position or to retain the enema solution. *Comments:*	☐	☐	☐	
3. Assess the client's mental state, including ability to understand and cooperate with the procedure, the client's knowledge level regarding the procedure, and any preexisting fears the client may have regarding the procedure. *Comments:*	☐	☐	☐	
Planning/Expected Outcomes				
1. The client's rectum will be free of feces and flatus. *Comments:*	☐	☐	☐	
2. The client will experience a minimum of trauma and embarrassment from the procedure. *Comments:*	☐	☐	☐	
Implementation				
Administering an Enema				
1. Check client's identification band and explain procedure before beginning. Wash hands. *Comments:*	☐	☐	☐	
2. Assess client's understanding of the procedure. Provide privacy. *Comments:*	☐	☐	☐	

continued on the following page

continued from the previous page

Procedure 29-29	Able to Perform	Able to Perform with Assistance	Unable to Perform	Initials and Date
3. Apply gloves. *Comments:*	☐	☐	☐	
4. Prepare equipment. *Comments:*	☐	☐	☐	
5. Place absorbent pad on bed under the client. Assist client into left lateral position with right leg flexed as sharply as possible. If there is a question regarding the client's ability to hold the solution, place a bedpan on the bed nearby. *Comments:*	☐	☐	☐	
6. Actions 6–12 are specific instructions for administering a large-volume cleansing enema. Enemas administered to adults are usually given at 105°–110° F (40.5°–43° C), and those administered to children are usually administered at 100° F (37.7° C). Solution should be at least body temperature to prevent cramping and discomfort. *Comments:*	☐	☐	☐	
7. Pour solution into the bag or bucket; add water if needed. Open clamp and prime tubing. Clamp tubing when primed. *Comments:*	☐	☐	☐	
8. Lubricate 5 cm (2 inches) of the rectal tube unless the tube is prelubricated. *Comments:*	☐	☐	☐	
9. Hold the enema container level with the rectum. Ask the client take a deep breath. Simultaneously, slowly and smoothly insert rectal tube into rectum approximately 7–10 cm (3–4 inches) in an adult. The tube should be inserted beyond the internal sphincter. Aim the rectal tube toward the client's umbilicus. *Comments:*	☐	☐	☐	
10. Raise the solution container and open clamp. (If using enema set, gently squeeze the container holding solution.) The solution should be 30–45 cm (12–18 inches) above the rectum for an adult and 7.5 cm (3 inches) above the rectum for an infant. *Comments:*	☐	☐	☐	
11. Slowly administer the fluid. *Comments:*	☐	☐	☐	

Procedure 29-29	Able to Perform	Able to Perform with Assistance	Unable to Perform	Initials and Date
12. When solution has been completely administered or when the client cannot hold any more fluid, clamp the tubing, remove the rectal tube, and dispose of it properly. *Comments:*	☐	☐	☐	
13. Actions 13–18 are specific instructions for administering a small-volume prepackaged enema. Remove packaged enema from packaging. Be familiar with any special instructions included with the enema. The packaged enema may be stood in a basin of warm water to warm the fluid before use. *Comments:*	☐	☐	☐	
14. Remove the protective cap from the nozzle and inspect the nozzle for lubrication. If the lubrication is not adequate, add more. *Comments:*	☐	☐	☐	
15. Squeeze the container gently to remove any air and to prime the nozzle. *Comments:*	☐	☐	☐	
16. Have the client take a deep breath. Simultaneously, gently insert the enema nozzle into the anus, pointing the nozzle toward the umbilicus. *Comments:*	☐	☐	☐	
17. Squeeze the container until all the solution is instilled and remove the nozzle from the anus. *Comments:*	☐	☐	☐	
18. Dispose of the empty container in an appropriate receptacle. *Comments:*	☐	☐	☐	
19. Clean lubricant, solution, and any feces from the anus with toilet tissue. *Comments:*	☐	☐	☐	
20. Have the client continue to lie on the left side for the prescribed length of time. A client may need to expel a large-volume cleansing enema soon after administration. Usually a client can hold a small-volume prepackaged enema the recommended minutes mentioned on the package. *Comments:*	☐	☐	☐	

continued on the following page

continued from the previous page

Procedure 29-29	Able to Perform	Able to Perform with Assistance	Unable to Perform	Initials and Date
21. When the client has retained the enema for the prescribed amount of time, assist the client to the bedside commode, toilet, or bedpan. If the client is using the bathroom, instruct client not to flush the toilet when finished. *Comments:*	☐	☐	☐	
22. When the client is finished expelling the enema, assist with cleaning the perineal area if needed. *Comments:*	☐	☐	☐	
23. Return the client to a comfortable position. Place a clean, dry protective pad under the client to catch any solution or feces that may continue to be expelled. *Comments:*	☐	☐	☐	
24. Remove gloves and wash hands. *Comments:*	☐	☐	☐	
Evaluation				
1. The client's rectum is free of feces or flatus. *Comments:*	☐	☐	☐	
2. The client experienced a minimum of trauma and embarrassment from the procedure. *Comments:*	☐	☐	☐	

Checklist for Procedure 29-30   Measuring Intake and Output

Name _____ Date _____

School _____

Instructor _____

Course _____

Procedure 29-30 Measuring Intake and Output	Able to Perform	Able to Perform with Assistance	Unable to Perform	Initials and Date
Assessment				
1. Assess the client's risk factors for fluid overload, such as congestive heart failure, renal failure, or ascites. *Comments:*	☐	☐	☐	
2. Determine if the client is receiving fluids or medications that predispose to fluid overload, such as large amounts of IV fluids or steroid therapy. *Comments:*	☐	☐	☐	
3. Assess the client's risk factors for fluid loss, such as diaphoresis, rapid respirations, diarrhea, gastric solution, blood loss, or wound drainage. *Comments:*	☐	☐	☐	
4. Determine if the client's urine output is in excess of fluid intake. *Comments:*	☐	☐	☐	
5. Assess the client's ability to understand and cooperate with intake and output measurement. *Comments:*	☐	☐	☐	
Planning/Expected Outcomes				
1. The client's fluid intake and output (I&O) will be accurately measured and recorded. *Comments:*	☐	☐	☐	
2. The client will participate in the recording of fluid I&O if possible. *Comments:*	☐	☐	☐	

continued on the following page

continued from the previous page

Procedure 29-30	Able to Perform	Able to Perform with Assistance	Unable to Perform	Initials and Date
Implementation				
Intake				
1. Check client's identification band and explain procedure before beginning. Wash hands. *Comments:*	☐	☐	☐	
2. Explain the rules of I&O record. The client must void into bedpan, urinal, or "hat" in toilet for collecting urine, not in toilet. Toilet tissue is disposed of in plastic-lined container, not in the urine collecting devices. *Comments:*	☐	☐	☐	
Intake				
3. Measure all oral fluids in accord with agency policy. Record all IV fluids as they are infused. *Comments:*	☐	☐	☐	
4. Record time and amount of all fluid intake in the designated space on bedside form (oral, tube feedings, IV fluids). *Comments:*	☐	☐	☐	
5. Transfer 8-hour total fluid intake from bedside I&O record to graphic sheet or 24-hour I&O record on the client's chart or client's computer record. *Comments:*	☐	☐	☐	
6. Record all fluid intake in the appropriate column of the 24-hour record, or enter intake appropriately in the computer record. *Comments:*	☐	☐	☐	
7. Complete 24-hour intake record by adding all 8-hour totals, or check that the computer has calculated data appropriately. *Comments:*	☐	☐	☐	
Output				
8. Wash hands and apply nonsterile gloves. *Comments:*	☐	☐	☐	
9. Empty urinal, bedpan, or Foley drainage bag into graduated container or commode "hat." *Comments:*	☐	☐	☐	

continued from the previous page

Procedure 29-30	Able to Perform	Able to Perform with Assistance	Unable to Perform	Initials and Date
10. Remove gloves and wash hands. *Comments:*	☐	☐	☐	
11. Record time and amount of output (urine, drainage from nasogastric tube, drainage tubes) on I&O record. *Comments:*	☐	☐	☐	
12. Transfer 8-hour output totals to graphic sheet or 24-hour I&O record on the client's chart or client's computerized record. *Comments:*	☐	☐	☐	
13. Complete 24-hour output record by totaling all 8-hour totals, or check that the computer has calculated data appropriately. *Comments:*	☐	☐	☐	
14. Wash hands. *Comments:*	☐	☐	☐	
Evaluation				
1. The client's fluid I&O were accurately measured and recorded. *Comments:*	☐	☐	☐	
2. The client participated in the recording of fluid I&O to the best of his or her ability. *Comments:*	☐	☐	☐	
3. Any abnormal findings were noted and reported to the client's health care provider. *Comments:*	☐	☐	☐	

Checklist for Procedure 29-31   Urine Collection—Closed Drainage System

Name _____ Date _____

School _____

Instructor _____

Course _____

Procedure 29-31 Urine Collection—Closed Drainage System	Able to Perform	Able to Perform with Assistance	Unable to Perform	Initials and Date
Assessment				
1. Identify the purpose of the urine test. *Comments:*	☐	☐	☐	
2. Assess the client's understanding of the test. *Comments:*	☐	☐	☐	
3. Identify the type of collecting tubing attached to the indwelling catheter. *Comments:*	☐	☐	☐	
Planning/Expected Outcomes				
1. Client understands the reason for the specimen. *Comments:*	☐	☐	☐	
2. Specimen is obtained in the proper container in a timely manner. *Comments:*	☐	☐	☐	
3. Specimen will remain uncontaminated. *Comments:*	☐	☐	☐	
Implementation				
1. Check client's identification band and explain procedure before beginning. Wash hands. *Comments:*	☐	☐	☐	
2. Check health care provider's order. *Comments:*	☐	☐	☐	
3. Provide privacy. *Comments:*	☐	☐	☐	

continued on the following page

continued from the previous page

Procedure 29-31	Able to Perform	Able to Perform with Assistance	Unable to Perform	Initials and Date
4. Check for urine in the tubing. *Comments:*	☐	☐	☐	
5. If more urine is needed, clamp the tubing using a nonserrated clamp or a rubber band for 10–15 minutes. *Comments:*	☐	☐	☐	
6. Put on clean gloves. *Comments:*	☐	☐	☐	
7. Clean sample port with an alcohol or povidone-iodine swab. *Comments:*	☐	☐	☐	
8. Insert sterile needle or plastic cannula of syringe into the sample port of catheter at a 45-degree angle and withdraw 10 ml of urine. *Comments:*	☐	☐	☐	
9. Put urine into sterile container and close tightly, taking care not to contaminate the lid of the container. *Comments:*	☐	☐	☐	
10. Place needle and syringe into sharps container. Never recap contaminated needle. *Comments:*	☐	☐	☐	
11. Remove clamp and rearrange tubing, avoiding dependent loops. *Comments:*	☐	☐	☐	
12. Label specimen container, put it in doubled plastic bag, and send to the laboratory. *Comments:*	☐	☐	☐	
13. Wash hands. *Comments:*	☐	☐	☐	
Evaluation				
1. The client understands the reason for the specimen. *Comments:*	☐	☐	☐	

Procedure 29-31	Able to Perform	Able to Perform with Assistance	Unable to Perform	Initials and Date
2. The specimen was obtained in the proper container in a timely manner. *Comments:*	☐	☐	☐	
3. The specimen remained uncontaminated. *Comments:*	☐	☐	☐	

Checklist for Procedure 29-32 Urine Collection—Clean Catch, Female/Male

Name _____ Date _____

School _____

Instructor _____

Course _____

Procedure 29-32 Urine Collection—Clean Catch, Female/Male	Able to Perform	Able to Perform with Assistance	Unable to Perform	Initials and Date
Assessment				
1. Evaluate the client's ability to obtain a clean-catch specimen. *Comments:*	☐	☐	☐	
2. Assess the presence of signs and symptoms of urinary tract infections or other abnormalities. *Comments:*	☐	☐	☐	
Planning/Expected Outcomes				
1. The client will be able to obtain a clean, midstream specimen. *Comments:*	☐	☐	☐	
2. The client will have absence of urinary abnormalities, such as burning, tingling, pain upon urination, or inability to control stream. *Comments:*	☐	☐	☐	
3. The client will understand procedure. *Comments:*	☐	☐	☐	
Implementation				
1. Check client's identification band and explain procedure before beginning. Check orders and assess need for procedure. *Comments:*	☐	☐	☐	
2. Gather equipment. *Comments:*	☐	☐	☐	
3. Assess the client's ability to complete the procedure, including understanding, mobility, and balance. *Comments:*	☐	☐	☐	

continued on the following page

continued from the previous page

Procedure 29-32	Able to Perform	Able to Perform with Assistance	Unable to Perform	Initials and Date
4. If nurse is to perform procedure, wash hands and apply gloves. If the client performs procedure, instruct client to wash hands before and after the procedure. If client wishes, provide a pair of gloves. *Comments:*	☐	☐	☐	
5. Provide privacy. *Comments:*	☐	☐	☐	
6. Using sterile procedure, open kit or towelettes. Open sterile container, placing the lid with sterile side up on a firm surface. *Comments:*	☐	☐	☐	
7. Female client: Sit with legs separated on the toilet. Use thumb and forefinger to separate labia or have client separate labia with fingers. With the labia separated, use a downward stroke (from the top of the labia down toward the rectal area) to cleanse each side of the labia and the urethral opening. Use a new towelette each time. Discard the towelette. *Comments:*	☐	☐	☐	
8. Male client: Stand in front of toilet. Pull back the foreskin (if present in uncircumcised male) and clean with a single stroke around meatus and glans. Use a circular motion, starting with the head of the penis at the urethral opening, moving down the glans shaft. Discard the towelette and repeat the procedure with another towelette, keeping the foreskin retracted. Wipe the head of the penis three times using a circular motion. Use a new towelette each time. *Comments:*	☐	☐	☐	
9. Ask the client to begin to urinate into the toilet. After the urine stream starts with good flow, place the collection cup under the stream of urine. Avoid touching the skin with the container. Fill the container with 30–60 mL of urine and remove the container before urination ceases. Wipe with toilet paper. *Comments:*	☐	☐	☐	
10. Place the sterile lid back onto the container and close tightly. Clean and dry the outside of the container with a towelette. Wash hands. Label and enclose in a double plastic biohazard bag, and follow facility policy for transporting specimen to the laboratory. *Comments:*	☐	☐	☐	

Procedure 29-32	Able to Perform	Able to Perform with Assistance	Unable to Perform	Initials and Date
11. Remove and dispose of gloves and wash hands. *Comments:*	☐	☐	☐	
Evaluation				
1. Clean midstream specimen was obtained. *Comments:*	☐	☐	☐	
2. The client understood procedure. *Comments:*	☐	☐	☐	
3. The client had no complaints associated with urination, such as burning, pain, or inability to initiate urination. *Comments:*	☐	☐	☐	

Checklist for Procedure 29-33 Collecting Nose, Throat, and Sputum Specimens

Name _____ Date _____

School _____

Instructor _____

Course _____

Procedure 29-33 Collecting Nose, Throat, and Sputum Specimens	Able to Perform	Able to Perform with Assistance	Unable to Perform	Initials and Date
Assessment				
1. Assess the client's understanding of the purpose of the procedure. *Comments:*	☐	☐	☐	
2. Assess the type of nasal or sinus drainage. *Comments:*	☐	☐	☐	
3. Review the health care provider's orders for the cultures requested. *Comments:*	☐	☐	☐	
4. Assess the client for postnasal drip, sinus headache, tenderness, nasal congestion, or sore throat. *Comments:*	☐	☐	☐	
5. Identify whether the client has received recent antimicrobials and obtain a specimen before treatment, if possible. *Comments:*	☐	☐	☐	
Planning/Expected Outcomes				
1. An adequate specimen will be obtained and sent to the laboratory. *Comments:*	☐	☐	☐	
2. The procedure will be performed with a minimum of trauma to the client. *Comments:*	☐	☐	☐	
Implementation				
1. Check client's identification band and explain procedure before beginning. Wash hands and put on clean gloves. *Comments:*	☐	☐	☐	

continued on the following page

continued from the previous page

Procedure 29-33	Able to Perform	Able to Perform with Assistance	Unable to Perform	Initials and Date
2. Ask the client to sit erect in bed or on chair facing the nurse. *Comments:*	☐	☐	☐	
3. Prepare a sterile swab for use by loosening the top of the container. *Comments:*	☐	☐	☐	
Collect Throat Culture				
4. Ask the client to tilt head backward, open mouth, and say "ah." *Comments:*	☐	☐	☐	
5. Depress the lateral anterior one-third of tongue with a tongue blade for better visualization. *Comments:*	☐	☐	☐	
6. Insert swab without touching cheek, lips, teeth, or tongue. *Comments:*	☐	☐	☐	
7. Swab tonsillar area from side to side in a quick, gentle motion. *Comments:*	☐	☐	☐	
8. Withdraw swab without touching adjacent structures and place in culture tube. Crush ampule at bottom of tube and push swab into liquid medium. *Comments:*	☐	☐	☐	
9. Secure top to culture tube and label with the client's name. *Comments:*	☐	☐	☐	
10. Discard tongue depressor. Remove gloves and discard. Wash hands. *Comments:*	☐	☐	☐	
Collect Nose Culture				
11. Instruct the client to blow nose. Check nostrils for patency with penlight. *Comments:*	☐	☐	☐	

Procedure 29-33	Able to Perform	Able to Perform with Assistance	Unable to Perform	Initials and Date
12. Ask the client to occlude one nostril, then the other, and exhale. *Comments:*	☐	☐	☐	
13. Ask the client to tilt head back. *Comments:*	☐	☐	☐	
14. Insert swab into nostril until it reaches the inflamed mucosa and rotate the swab. *Comments:*	☐	☐	☐	
15. Withdraw the swab without touching adjacent structures and place in culture tube. Crush ampule at bottom of tube and push swab into liquid medium. *Comments:*	☐	☐	☐	
16. Secure top to culture tube and label with the client's name. *Comments:*	☐	☐	☐	
17. Remove gloves and discard. Wash hands. *Comments:*	☐	☐	☐	
Collection of Nasopharyngeal Culture				
18. Follow Actions 11–17 except use a swab on a flexible wire that can reach the nasopharynx via the nose. *Comments:*	☐	☐	☐	
Collecting a Sputum Culture				
19. Explain to the client that the specimen must be sputum, coughed up from the lungs. *Comments:*	☐	☐	☐	
20. Have a sterile specimen cup ready for the sample and some tissues at hand. *Comments:*	☐	☐	☐	
21. Have the client take several deep breaths and then cough deeply. *Comments:*	☐	☐	☐	
22. Have the client expectorate the sputum into the sterile cup without touching the inside of the cup. *Comments:*	☐	☐	☐	

continued on the following page

continued from the previous page

Procedure 29-33	Able to Perform	Able to Perform with Assistance	Unable to Perform	Initials and Date
23. Place the lid on the specimen container without touching the inside of the lid or the container. *Comments:*	☐	☐	☐	
24. Provide the client with tissue and make him or her comfortable. *Comments:*	☐	☐	☐	
Alternative Sputum Collection Method **(used if the client is unable to expectorate an adequate sample)**				
25. Obtain a sterile suction catheter and an in-line sputum collection container. *Comments:*	☐	☐	☐	
26. Provide the client with warm humidified air for about 20 minutes if it is not contraindicated by the client's condition. *Comments:*	☐	☐	☐	
27. Hook the sputum collector up to suction tubing and a suction device. Hook the suction catheter to the sputum collector. *Comments:*	☐	☐	☐	
28. If the client is able to cooperate, have him or her take several deep breaths and cough. *Comments:*	☐	☐	☐	
29. As the client is coughing up sputum, carefully insert the catheter either orally or nasopharyngeally into the back of the client's throat and suction the sputum into the specimen container. *Comments:*	☐	☐	☐	
30. Safely dispose of the suction catheter. *Comments:*	☐	☐	☐	
31. Close the specimen container. *Comments:*	☐	☐	☐	
32. Provide tissues or other measures for client comfort. *Comments:*	☐	☐	☐	
33. Wash hands. *Comments:*	☐	☐	☐	

Procedure 29-33	Able to Perform	Able to Perform with Assistance	Unable to Perform	Initials and Date
34. Label each specimen with client's name and send to the laboratory. *Comments:*	☐	☐	☐	
Evaluation				
1. An adequate specimen was obtained. *Comments:*	☐	☐	☐	
2. The procedure was performed with a minimum of trauma to the client. *Comments:*	☐	☐	☐	

Checklist for Procedure 29-34   Collecting a Stool Specimen

Name _____ Date _____

School _____

Instructor _____

Course _____

Procedure 29-34 Collecting a Stool Specimen	Able to Perform	Able to Perform with Assistance	Unable to Perform	Initials and Date
Assessment				
1. Assess the client's or family member's understanding of the need for this test. *Comments:*	☐	☐	☐	
2. Assess the client's ability to cooperate with the procedure. *Comments:*	☐	☐	☐	
3. Assess the client's medical history for bleeding or gastrointestinal (GI) disorders. *Comments:*	☐	☐	☐	
4. Assess any medications the client receives that can cause GI bleeding, such as anticoagulants, steroids, or acetylsalicylic acid. *Comments:*	☐	☐	☐	
Planning/Expected Outcomes				
1. The client will understand the purpose of the test. *Comments:*	☐	☐	☐	
2. The client will be able to collect the specimen, or allow the specimen to be collected. *Comments:*	☐	☐	☐	
3. The test will be conducted properly and the results recorded. *Comments:*	☐	☐	☐	
Implementation				
1. Check client's identification band and explain procedure before beginning. Wash hands and apply clean gloves. *Comments:*	☐	☐	☐	

continued on the following page

continued from the previous page

Procedure 29-34	Able to Perform	Able to Perform with Assistance	Unable to Perform	Initials and Date
2. Assist the client as needed to bedside commode or toilet. Have client void before moving bowels. Prepare for specimen collection. If client is not ambulatory, use a bedpan. For the toilet, use a "hat." Place "hat" in the back section of toilet to collect stool specimen, and the front section to collect urine specimen. *Comments:*	☐	☐	☐	
3. Instruct the client not to contaminate the specimen with urine, vaginal discharge, or toilet tissue. *Comments:*	☐	☐	☐	
4. Ask the client to notify you as soon as the specimen is available. *Comments:*	☐	☐	☐	
5. Assist the client with hygiene, help the client back to bed (as required), and ensure client comfort before turning attention to specimen. *Comments:*	☐	☐	☐	
6. Apply gloves; wear gown if client is on isolation or at risk for infectious stool, such as vancomycin-resistant enterococcus (VRE). *Comments:*	☐	☐	☐	
7. Assess stool color, consistency, odor and presence or absence of visible blood or mucus. *Comments:*	☐	☐	☐	
8. Using one or two tongue blades, transfer a representative sample of stool to the specimen card or container, taking care not to contaminate the outside of the container (or the inside of a sterile specimen cup). If using a culture swab, swab in a representative area of stool, particularly if any purulent material is visible. Check with laboratory regarding the volume of stool needed for a particular test. *Comments:*	☐	☐	☐	
9. Close the card, place the lid on the container, or place the swab in the culture tube (according to agency policy) as soon as specimen is collected. *Comments:*	☐	☐	☐	

Procedure 29-34	Able to Perform	Able to Perform with Assistance	Unable to Perform	Initials and Date
10. Place the specimen container in a plastic biohazard bag for transport to the laboratory after proper labeling is done according to agency policy. Be careful not to contaminate the outside of the bag. Provide requisition for test according to agency policy. *Comments:*	☐	☐	☐	
11. Dispose of rest of stool according to agency policy. *Comments:*	☐	☐	☐	
12. Remove gloves and wash hands. *Comments:*	☐	☐	☐	
13. Send specimen to the laboratory immediately. *Comments:*	☐	☐	☐	
Evaluation				
1. Specimen collected and transported to the laboratory. *Comments:*	☐	☐	☐	
2. Note color, character, and consistency of stool. *Comments:*	☐	☐	☐	
3. Client is able to explain the rationale and procedure for the stool test. *Comments:*	☐	☐	☐	

Checklist for Procedure 29-35   Applying Velcro Abdominal Binders

Name _____ Date _____

School _____

Instructor _____

Course _____

Procedure 29-35 Applying Velcro Abdominal Binders	Able to Perform	Able to Perform with Assistance	Unable to Perform	Initials and Date
Assessment				
1. Assess the reason the binder is needed to determine the correct binder and correct placement. *Comments:*	☐	☐	☐	
2. Assess the client's skin condition for rashes, inflammation, open areas, or dressings. *Comments:*	☐	☐	☐	
3. Assess and measure the client to determine what size binder is needed. *Comments:*	☐	☐	☐	
4. Assess for any special circumstances that may affect the placement of the binder, such as dressings, tubing, catheters, or IV lines. *Comments:*	☐	☐	☐	
5. Assess the client's understanding of the procedure. *Comments:*	☐	☐	☐	
Planning/Expected Outcomes				
1. Binder will provide support for dressings or soft tissue. *Comments:*	☐	☐	☐	
2. Binder will not be too tight or compress the skin. *Comments:*	☐	☐	☐	
3. Client will assist in the placement of the binder as much as possible. *Comments:*	☐	☐	☐	

continued on the following page

continued from the previous page

Procedure 29-35	Able to Perform	Able to Perform with Assistance	Unable to Perform	Initials and Date
Implementation				
Abdominal Binders				
1. Check client's identification band and explain procedure before beginning. Wash hands. *Comments:*	☐	☐	☐	
2. Choose correct size binder. *Comments:*	☐	☐	☐	
3. Help the client into the proper position to place the binder. For abdominal Velcro binders, the client should lie supine and lift the hips; or alternatively, position the client on one side and roll the client onto binder. *Comments:*	☐	☐	☐	
4. Secure binder with Velcro. *Comments:*	☐	☐	☐	
5. Wash hands. *Comments:*	☐	☐	☐	
Evaluation				
1. Binder provides support for dressing or soft tissue. *Comments:*	☐	☐	☐	
2. Binder is not too tight and does not compress the skin. *Comments:*	☐	☐	☐	
3. Client assists in placement of the binder as much as possible. *Comments:*	☐	☐	☐	

Checklist for Procedure 29-36   Application of Restraints

Name _____ Date _____

School _____

Instructor _____

Course _____

Procedure 29-36 Application of Restraints	Able to Perform	Able to Perform with Assistance	Unable to Perform	Initials and Date
Assessment				
1. Assess the client's level of consciousness. *Comments:*	☐	☐	☐	
2. Assess the client's degree of orientation. *Comments:*	☐	☐	☐	
3. Assess the client's physical condition. *Comments:*	☐	☐	☐	
4. Assess the client's history for falls, accidents, confusion, agitation, or self-inflicted injury. *Comments:*	☐	☐	☐	
5. Assess the client's intent. *Comments:*	☐	☐	☐	
6. Assess need for restraints. Determine if the client's treatment plan requires and allows restraints, if orders are in place, and if hospital policies and laws are specified. *Comments:*	☐	☐	☐	
7. Assess client and family knowledge regarding the use of and rationale for restraints or protective devices. *Comments:*	☐	☐	☐	
Planning/Expected Outcomes				
1. The client will remain uninjured. *Comments:*	☐	☐	☐	
2. The client will not suffer injury or impairment from the restraints. *Comments:*	☐	☐	☐	

continued on the following page

continued from the previous page

Procedure 29-36	Able to Perform	Able to Perform with Assistance	Unable to Perform	Initials and Date
3. The client's therapeutic equipment will remain intact and functional. *Comments:*	☐	☐	☐	
4. Others will not be harmed by the client. *Comments:*	☐	☐	☐	
5. The client will be restrained just enough to prevent injury. *Comments:*	☐	☐	☐	
Implementation				
Chest Restraint 1. Check client's identification band and wash hands. Explain that for safety, the client will be wearing a jacket attached to the bed. *Comments:*	☐	☐	☐	
2. Place the restraint over the client's hospital gown or clothing. *Comments:*	☐	☐	☐	
3. Place the restraint on the client with the opening in the front. *Comments:*	☐	☐	☐	
4. Overlap the front pieces, threading the ties through the slot/loop on the front of the vest. *Comments:*	☐	☐	☐	
5. If the client is in bed, secure the ties to the movable part of the mattress frame with a half-knot or quick-release knot. *Comments:*	☐	☐	☐	
6. If the client is in a chair, cross the straps behind the back of the chair and secure the straps to the chair's lower legs, out of the client's reach. If it is a wheelchair, be sure the straps will not get caught in the wheels. *Comments:*	☐	☐	☐	
7. Step back and assess the client's overall safety. Be sure the restraint is loose enough not to be a hazard to the client but tight enough to restrict the client from getting up and harming him or herself. *Comments:*	☐	☐	☐	

Procedure 29-36	Able to Perform	Able to Perform with Assistance	Unable to Perform	Initials and Date
8. Wash hands. *Comments:*	☐	☐	☐	
Applying Wrist or Ankle Restraints				
1. Explain that you are placing a wrist or ankle band that will restrict movement. *Comments:*	☐	☐	☐	
2. Wrap the restraint around the wrist or ankle and fasten with Velcro grips. *Comments:*	☐	☐	☐	
3. Secure the restraint to the movable portion of the mattress frame with a half-knot ir quick-release knot. *Comments:*	☐	☐	☐	
4. Slip two fingers under the restraint to check for tightness. Restraint should be tight enough that the client cannot slip it off but loose enough that the neurovascular status of the client's extremity is not impaired. *Comments:*	☐	☐	☐	
5. Step back and assess the client's overall safety. Restraint should be loose enough not to be a hazard but tight enough to restrict the client from getting up and harming him or herself. *Comments:*	☐	☐	☐	
6. Place the call light within the client's reach. *Comments:*	☐	☐	☐	
7. Assess the client 15 minutes after the initiation of restraints or seclusion with special attention to the client's emotional status, safety of the restraint placement, and the client's neurovascular status. After 15 minutes, use clinical judgment or health care practitioner orders to establish a routine for assessing client's needs. A physician or health care practitioner must evaluate the client within 1 hour of the application of the restraint and write an order for restraint as deemed necessary. *Comments:*	☐	☐	☐	
8. Wash hands. *Comments:*	☐	☐	☐	

continued on the following page

continued from the previous page

Procedure 29-36	Able to Perform	Able to Perform with Assistance	Unable to Perform	Initials and Date
Evaluation				
1. Client remained uninjured. *Comments:*	☐	☐	☐	
2. Client has not suffered injury or impairment from the restraints. *Comments:*	☐	☐	☐	
3. Client's therapeutic equipment remained intact and functional. *Comments:*	☐	☐	☐	
4. Others have not been harmed by the client. *Comments:*	☐	☐	☐	
5. Client is restrained just enough to prevent injury. *Comments:*	☐	☐	☐	

Checklist for Procedure 29-37   Performing the Heimlich Maneuver

Name _____ Date _____

School _____

Instructor _____

Course _____

Procedure 29-37 **Performing the Heimlich Maneuver**	Able to Perform	Able to Perform with Assistance	Unable to Perform	Initials and Date
Assessment				
1. Assess air exchange. Assess for complete or partial foreign body obstruction. *Comments:*	☐	☐	☐	
2. Establish airway obstruction. Check for universal sign of airway obstruction, the inability to talk or breathe, cyanosis, and the progression to an unconscious state. *Comments:*	☐	☐	☐	
3. In a pediatric client, differentiate between infection and airway obstruction. *Comments:*	☐	☐	☐	
Planning/Expected Outcomes				
1. The client's clinical status will improve. *Comments:*	☐	☐	☐	
2. The client's gas exchange will improve. *Comments:*	☐	☐	☐	
3. The client will experience minimal discomfort during the Heimlich maneuver or other method of airway clearance. *Comments:*	☐	☐	☐	
4. The client will not experience complications related to airway obstruction/hypoxia. *Comments:*	☐	☐	☐	
Implementation				
Foreign Body Obstruction—All Clients				
1. Assess airway for complete or partial blockage. *Comments:*	☐	☐	☐	

continued on the following page

continued from the previous page

Procedure 29-37	Able to Perform	Able to Perform with Assistance	Unable to Perform	Initials and Date
2. Encourage attempts to cough and breathe. *Comments:*	☐	☐	☐	
3. Activate emergency response assistance. *Comments:*	☐	☐	☐	
Conscious Adult Client—Sitting or Standing (Heimlich Maneuver)				
4. Stand behind the client and wrap your arms around the client's waist. *Comments:*	☐	☐	☐	
5. Make a fist with one hand and grasp it with your other hand, placing the thumb side of the fist against the client's abdomen. The fist is placed midline, below the xiphoid process and lower margins of the rib cage and above the navel. *Comments:*	☐	☐	☐	
6. Perform a quick upward thrust into the client's abdomen; each thrust is separate and distinct. *Comments:*	☐	☐	☐	
7. Repeat this process 6–10 times until the client either expels the foreign body or loses consciousness. *Comments:*	☐	☐	☐	
Unconscious Adult Client or Adult Client Who Becomes Unconscious				
8. Repeat Actions 1–3. *Comments:*	☐	☐	☐	
9. Position the client supine, kneel astride the client's abdomen. *Comments:*	☐	☐	☐	
10. Place the heel of one hand midline, below the xiphoid process and lower margin of the rib cage and above the navel. Place the second hand on top of the first hand. *Comments:*	☐	☐	☐	
11. Perform a quick upward thrust into the diaphragm, repeating 6 to 10 times. *Comments:*	☐	☐	☐	

Procedure 29-37	Able to Perform	Able to Perform with Assistance	Unable to Perform	Initials and Date
12. Perform a finger sweep. Use one hand to grasp the lower jaw and tongue between your thumb and fingers and lift; using the index finger of the other hand, do a finger sweep to remove any foreign body that can be easily seen and removed. *Comments:*	☐	☐	☐	
13. Open the client's airway and attempt ventilation. *Comments:*	☐	☐	☐	
14. Continue sequence of Heimlich maneuver, finger sweep, and rescue breathing as long as necessary. *Comments:*	☐	☐	☐	
Airway Obstruction—Infants and Small Children				
15. Differentiate between infection and airway obstruction. *Comments:*	☐	☐	☐	
Infant Airway Obstruction				
16. Straddle infant over your forearm in the prone position with the head lower than the trunk. Support the infant's head positioning a hand around the jaws and chest. *Comments:*	☐	☐	☐	
17. Deliver five back blows between the infant's shoulder blades. *Comments:*	☐	☐	☐	
18. Keeping the infant's head down, place the free hand on the infant's back and turn the infant over, supporting the back of the infant with your hand and thigh. *Comments:*	☐	☐	☐	
19. With your free hand, deliver five thrusts in the same manner as infant external cardiac compressions. *Comments:*	☐	☐	☐	
20. Assess for a foreign body in an unconscious infant and utilize the finger sweep only if a foreign body is visualized. *Comments:*	☐	☐	☐	
21. Open airway and assess for respiration. If respirations are absent, attempt rescue breathing. Assess for the rise and fall of the chest; if not seen, reposition infant and attempt rescue breathing again. *Comments:*	☐	☐	☐	

continued on the following page

continued from the previous page

Procedure 29-37	Able to Perform	Able to Perform with Assistance	Unable to Perform	Initials and Date
22. Repeat the entire sequence as long as necessary. *Comments:*	☐	☐	☐	
Small Child—Airway Obstruction (Conscious, Standing or Sitting)				
23. Assess air exchange and encourage coughing and breathing. Provide reassurance to the child that you are there to help. *Comments:*	☐	☐	☐	
24. Ask the child if he or she is choking. If the response is affirmative, follow the steps outlined below. If the child has poor air exchange (and infection has been ruled out), initiate the following steps: • Stand behind the child with your arms wrapped around his or her waist and quickly administer 6–10 subdiaphragmatic abdominal thrusts. • Continue until foreign object is expelled or the child becomes unconscious. *Comments:*	☐	☐	☐	
Small Child—Airway Obstruction (Unconscious)				
25. Position the child supine and kneel at the child's feet. Gently deliver five subdiaphragmatic abdominal thrusts. *Comments:*	☐	☐	☐	
26. Open airway. Perform a finger sweep only if a foreign body is visualized. *Comments:*	☐	☐	☐	
27. If breathing is absent, begin rescue breathing. If the chest does not rise, reposition the child and attempt rescue breathing again. *Comments:*	☐	☐	☐	
28. Repeat this sequence as long as necessary. *Comments:*	☐	☐	☐	
29. Wash hands. *Comments:*	☐	☐	☐	
Evaluation				
1. Client demonstrates improved clinical status as evidenced by airway clearance or establishment of a patent airway. *Comments:*	☐	☐	☐	

Procedure 29-37	Able to Perform	Able to Perform with Assistance	Unable to Perform	Initials and Date
2. Client demonstrates improved gas exchange as evidenced by absence of signs and symptoms of partial or complete airway obstruction. *Comments:*	☐	☐	☐	
3. Client experienced minimal discomfort during Heimlich maneuver or other method of airway clearance. *Comments:*	☐	☐	☐	
4. Client did not experience complications related to airway obstruction or hypoxia. *Comments:*	☐	☐	☐	

Checklist for Procedure 29-38 Performing Cardiopulmonary Resuscitation (CPR)

Name _____ Date _____

School _____

Instructor _____

Course _____

Procedure 29-38 Performing Cardiopulmonary Resuscitation (CPR)	Able to Perform	Able to Perform with Assistance	Unable to Perform	Initials and Date
Assessment				
1. Assess responsiveness and level of consciousness by gently shaking or tapping the client while shouting, "Are you OK?" *Comments:*	☐	☐	☐	
2. Assess the amount and abilities of any available assistance. CPR cannot be performed indefinitely by a single individual. *Comments:*	☐	☐	☐	
3. Assess the client's position. If needed, reposition in the client supine on a flat surface. *Comments:*	☐	☐	☐	
4. Assess respiratory status by looking for the chest to rise and fall, listening for air exchange, and feeling for the presence of air movement. *Comments:*	☐	☐	☐	
5. Assess circulatory status by using carotid or brachial pulse points. *Comments:*	☐	☐	☐	
Planning/Expected Outcomes				
1. The client will experience improved clinical status. *Comments:*	☐	☐	☐	
2. Client does not experience negative sequela related to hypoxic event. *Comments:*	☐	☐	☐	
3. Client does not have damage inflicted by incorrect positioning for CPR. *Comments:*	☐	☐	☐	
4. CPR will be terminated appropriately. *Comments:*	☐	☐	☐	

continued on the following page

continued from the previous page

Procedure 29-38	Able to Perform	Able to Perform with Assistance	Unable to Perform	Initials and Date
Implementation				
CPR: One Rescuer—Adult, Adolescent				
1. Assess responsiveness by tapping or gently shaking while shouting "Are you OK?" *Comments:*	☐	☐	☐	
2. Activate emergency medical system. In the hospital or clinical setting, follow institutional protocol. In the community or home environment, activate the local emergency response system. *Comments:*	☐	☐	☐	
3. Position client in a supine position on a hard, flat surface. Use caution when positioning a client with a possible head or neck injury. *Comments:*	☐	☐	☐	
4. Apply appropriate body substance isolation items, if available. *Comments:*	☐	☐	☐	
5. Position self. Face the client on your knees parallel to the client, next to the head, to begin to assess the airway and breathing status. *Comments:*	☐	☐	☐	
6. Open airway using the head-tilt/chin-lift or jaw thrust methods. In the event of a suspected head or neck injury, this is modified and the jaw thrust is used without head extension. If available, insert oral airway. *Comments:*	☐	☐	☐	
7. Assess for respirations. Look, listen, and feel for air movement (3–5 seconds). *Comments:*	☐	☐	☐	
8. If respirations are absent: • Occlude nostrils with the thumb and index finger of the hand on the forehead that is tilting the head back. • Form a seal over the client's facemask using either your mouth or the appropriate respiratory assist device and give two full breaths. • Mouth-to-nose ventilation may be used. *Comments:*	☐	☐	☐	

Procedure 29-38	Able to Perform	Able to Perform with Assistance	Unable to Perform	Initials and Date
9. Assess for the rise and fall of the chest: • If present, continue to Action 10. • If absent, assess for excessive oral secretions, vomit, airway obstruction, or improper positioning. *Comments:*	☐	☐	☐	
10. Palpate the carotid pulse: • If present, continue rescue breathing at a rate of 12 breaths/min. • If absent, begin external cardiac compressions. *Comments:*	☐	☐	☐	
11. Cardiac compressions: • Maintain a position on knees parallel to the client's sternum. • Position hands for compressions. • Extend or interlace fingers. • Keep arms straight and lock elbows. • Compress at the age-appropriate rate. • Ventilate client as described in Action 8. *Comments:*	☐	☐	☐	
12. Maintain the compression rate, for approximately 100 times per minute, interjecting 2 ventilations after every 20 compressions. *Comments:*	☐	☐	☐	
13. Reassess the client after four cycles. *Comments:*	☐	☐	☐	
CPR: Two Rescuers—Adult, Adolescent 14. Follow Actions 1–13 with the following changes: • Rescuers are positioned on opposite sides of the client. • The rescuer at the trunk performs cardiac compressions and maintains the verbal count. This is rescuer 1. • The rescuer positioned at the head monitors respirations, assesses pulse, establishes an airway, and performs rescue breathing at a rate of 10–12 breaths/minute. This is rescuer 2. • Maintain the compression rate for approximately 100 times per minute, interjecting two ventilations after every 15 compressions. • Rescuer 2 palpates the carotid pulse with each chest compression during the first full minute.				

continued on the following page

continued from the previous page

Procedure 29-38	Able to Perform	Able to Perform with Assistance	Unable to Perform	Initials and Date
• Rescuer 2 is responsible for calling a change. Rescuers should change every 2 minutes or 5 cycles of CPR (1 cycle of CPR = 30 compressions; 2 breaths). Rescuer 2 follows this protocol. • Rescuer 1 calls for a change and completes the 15 chest compressions. • Rescuer 2 administers two breaths and then moves to a position parallel to the client's sternum and assumes the proper hand position. • Resucer 1 moves to the rescue breathing position and checks the carotid pulse for 5 seconds. If cardiac arrest persists, rescuer 1 says "continue CPR" and delivers one breath. Rescuer 2 resumes cardiac compressions immediately after the breath. *Comments:*	☐	☐	☐	
CPR: One Rescuer—Child (1–onset of adolescence/puberty)				
15. Follow Actions 1, 3–7. *Comments:*	☐	☐	☐	
16. If respirations are absent, begin rescue breathing. Give two slow breaths (1–1 1/2 seconds/breath), pausing to take a breath in between. Use only the amount of air needed to make the chest rise. *Comments:*	☐	☐	☐	
17. Palpate the carotid pulse (5–10 seconds): • If present, ventilate at a rate of once every 3–5 seconds or 12–20 breaths per minute. • If absent, begin cardiac compressions. *Comments:*	☐	☐	☐	
18. Cardiac compressions: • Maintain a position on knees parallel to child's sternum. • Position the hands for compressions, placing one hand on the sternum. • At the end of every 30th compression, administer 2 ventilations. • Re-evaluate child after 20 cycles. If respirations are still absent, call 911. *Comments:*	☐	☐	☐	
CPR: One Rescuer—Infant (1–12 months)				
19. Follow Actions 1, 3–7. *Comments:*	☐	☐	☐	

Procedure 29-38	Able to Perform	Able to Perform with Assistance	Unable to Perform	Initials and Date
20. If respirations are absent, begin rescue breathing. • Avoid overextension of the infant's neck. • Place a small towel or diaper under the infant's shoulders or use a hand to support the neck. • Make a tight seal over both the infant's nose and mouth and gently administer artificial respirations. • Give two slow breaths (1 second per breath), pausing to take a breath in between. • Use only the amount of air needed to make the chest rise. *Comments:*	☐	☐	☐	
21. Assess circulatory status using the brachial pulse: • If a pulse is palpated, continue rescue breathing 12–20 times per minute or once every 3–5 seconds. • If a pulse is absent, begin cardiac compressions. *Comments:*	☐	☐	☐	
22. Cardiac compressions (infant 1–12 months): • Maintain a position parallel to the infant. • Place a small towel under the infant's shoulders/neck. • Position the hands for compressions. • Using the hand closest to the infant's feet, locate the intermammary line where it intersects the sternum. • Place the index finger 1 cm below this location on the sternum and place the middle finger next to the index finger. • Using these two fingers, compress in a downward motion, one third to one half the depth of the chest, at the rate of 100 times per minute. • Keep the other hand on the infant's forehead. • Re-evaluate infant after 20 cycles. If respirations still absent, call 911. *Comments:*	☐	☐	☐	
CPR: Two Rescuers—Child (1–onset of adolescence/puberty)				
23. Follow Action 14 for two rescuer CPR for adults with the following changes: • Utilize the child or infant procedure for chest compressions. • Change the ratio of compressions to ventilation to 15:2. • Deliver the ventilation on the upstroke of the third compression. *Comments:*	☐	☐	☐	
CPR: Neonate or Premature Infant				
24. Follow the infant guidelines except: • Encircle the chest with both hands. • Position thumbs over the midsternum.				

continued on the following page

continued from the previous page

Procedure 29-38	Able to Perform	Able to Perform with Assistance	Unable to Perform	Initials and Date
• Compress the midsternum with both thumbs. • Compress one third to one half the depth of the chest at a rate of 100–120 times per minute. *Comments:*	☐	☐	☐	
25. Demonstrate proper use of an automated external defibrillator (AED). • Use adult defibrillation pads for adults. Use the pediatric system for a child of 1 to 8 years, if available. • Use AED after 5 cycles of CPR on a child between 1 year and the onset of adolescence/puberty. • In hospital setting, use defibrillator as specified by institution protocol. • The defibrillator should be placed only by properly trained personnel. *Comments:*	☐	☐	☐	
Evaluation				
1. An open airway is maintained, as evidenced by the chest rise and fall. *Comments:*	☐	☐	☐	
2. Resistance and compliance of the client's lungs is felt. *Comments:*	☐	☐	☐	
3. Airway movement during expiration is felt and heard. *Comments:*	☐	☐	☐	
4. Circulation indicators, such as color, improve. *Comments:*	☐	☐	☐	
5. Client has return of spontaneous pulse and respirations. *Comments:*	☐	☐	☐	
6. Assist with transfer to hospital/advanced life-support unit. If CPR was unsuccessful, assist in notifying next of kin and providing psychosocial support. *Comments:*	☐	☐	☐	

Checklist for Procedure 29-39   Admitting a Client

Name _____ Date _____

School _____

Instructor _____

Course _____

Procedure 29-39 Admitting a Client	Able to Perform	Able to Perform with Assistance	Unable to Perform	Initials and Date
Assessment				
1. Assess the client's comfort level about being in a health care facility. Comments:	☐	☐	☐	
2. Assess client's physical and mental state. Comments:	☐	☐	☐	
3. Assess the client's knowledge of reason for admission. Comments:	☐	☐	☐	
Planning/Expected Outcomes				
1. The client will be comfortable in the health care facility. Comments:	☐	☐	☐	
2. The client will understand how to use the call bell system, bed controls, television, and telephone. Comments:	☐	☐	☐	
3. The client will adjust to facility routine. Comments:	☐	☐	☐	
Implementation				
1. Wash hands. Welcome the client to unit and introduce self by name and title. Ask client to state his or her name. Comments:	☐	☐	☐	
2. Orient client to room, nursing unit, education materials, and other information about the facility. Comments:	☐	☐	☐	
3. Provide privacy for the client to change. Comments:	☐	☐	☐	

continued on the following page

continued from the previous page

Procedure 29-39	Able to Perform	Able to Perform with Assistance	Unable to Perform	Initials and Date
4. Show client ID bracelet to double-check proper identification. Attach bracelet to wrist. Review drug allergies and attach allergy bracelet to same wrist. *Comments:*	☐	☐	☐	
5. Document and store the client's belongings and valuables according to agency policy. *Comments:*	☐	☐	☐	
6. Begin nursing assessment. *Comments:*	☐	☐	☐	
7. Perform any other actions as directed by agency policy. *Comments:*	☐	☐	☐	
Evaluation				
1. Client is comfortable in the health care facility. *Comments:*	☐	☐	☐	
2. Client uses the call bell system, bed controls, television, and telephone. *Comments:*	☐	☐	☐	
3. Client has adjusted to facility routine. *Comments:*	☐	☐	☐	

Checklist for Procedure 29-40   Transferring a Client

Name _____ Date _____

School _____

Instructor _____

Course _____

Procedure 29-40 Transferring a Client	Able to Perform	Able to Perform with Assistance	Unable to Perform	Initials and Date
Assessment				
1. Assess the client's knowledge and feelings about the transfer. *Comments:*	☐	☐	☐	
2. Assess which equipment is to be transferred with the client and that medications and client's personal belongings are ready to move. *Comments:*	☐	☐	☐	
3. Assess readiness of new unit to accept client. *Comments:*	☐	☐	☐	
Planning/Expected Outcomes				
1. Client will understand reason for transfer. *Comments:*	☐	☐	☐	
2. Client will be safely moved with needed equipment, medication, and all personal belongings. *Comments:*	☐	☐	☐	
3. Client's move will be communicated to appropriate departments for continuity of care. *Comments:*	☐	☐	☐	
Implementation				
1. Check client's identification band and wash hands. Check transfer orders. *Comments:*	☐	☐	☐	
2. Call nursing unit of new location to see if bed is ready and give report. *Comments:*	☐	☐	☐	

continued on the following page

continued from the previous page

Procedure 29-40	Able to Perform	Able to Perform with Assistance	Unable to Perform	Initials and Date
3. Explain the transfer to the client (and family, if appropriate). Answer questions. Allay anxieties about moving. *Comments:*	☐	☐	☐	
4. Review the valuables and belongings checklist completed on admission. Compare with belongings. *Comments:*	☐	☐	☐	
5. Gather records and any equipment that are transferred with the client according to agency policy. *Comments:*	☐	☐	☐	
6. Transfer client by appropriate vehicle. Accompany client to new unit. Transfer care to another staff member in person. Ensure call light is within reach of client or staff member in room before leaving client. *Comments:*	☐	☐	☐	
7. Document time of transfer and any other information required by agency policy. *Comments:*	☐	☐	☐	
8. Upon return to unit, notify appropriate personnel according to agency policy that the client has left the unit. Arrange for personnel to clean the bed and surroundings the client left. *Comments:*	☐	☐	☐	
Evaluation				
1. Client understood the reason for transferring to a new unit. *Comments:*	☐	☐	☐	
2. Client was safely moved, with needed equipment, medications, and all personal belongings. *Comments:*	☐	☐	☐	
3. Client's move was communicated to appropriate departments for continuity of care. *Comments:*	☐	☐	☐	

Checklist for Procedure 29-41   Discharging a Client

Name _____ Date _____

School _____

Instructor _____

Course _____

Procedure 29-41 **Discharging a Client**	Able to Perform	Able to Perform with Assistance	Unable to Perform	Initials and Date
Assessment				
1. Assess the client's feelings about being discharged. *Comments:*	☐	☐	☐	
2. Assess that family/home or other facility is prepared to receive the client. *Comments:*	☐	☐	☐	
3. Assess the client's or family's knowledge of care at home. *Comments:*	☐	☐	☐	
Planning/Expected Outcomes				
1. The client will complete discharge to another facility with no problems. *Comments:*	☐	☐	☐	
2. The client will feel confident about care at home. *Comments:*	☐	☐	☐	
Implementation				
1. Check client's identification band and wash hands. Check order for discharge. *Comments:*	☐	☐	☐	
Discharge to Another Facility				
2. Explain discharge to the client (and family, if appropriate). *Comments:*	☐	☐	☐	
3. Complete intra-agency transfer form, note medication doses, complete discharge summary, and prepare transfer paperwork, according to policy. *Comments:*	☐	☐	☐	

continued on the following page

continued from the previous page

Procedure 29-41	Able to Perform	Able to Perform with Assistance	Unable to Perform	Initials and Date
4. Notify receiving agency of impending transfer, provide report, and confirm ability to receive the client. *Comments:*	☐	☐	☐	
5. Arrange for transportation to the new facility. Call transportation company according to agency policy *Comments:*	☐	☐	☐	
6. Review valuables and belongings checklist completed on admission. Compare with belongings. *Comments:*	☐	☐	☐	
7. When personnel from the transportation company arrive, assist client transfer to stretcher or wheelchair. Provide transportation personnel with required information, such as client's DNR status, for transfer. See that client's belongings accompany client, along with and any required paperwork and equipment. *Comments:*	☐	☐	☐	
Discharge to Home				
8. Discuss discharge with the client (and family, if appropriate). Confirm discharge teaching has been done. Ask client if there are any questions about self-care at home. If so, follow up with appropriate personnel. *Comments:*	☐	☐	☐	
9. Review with client prescriptions, food/drug interactions, care of incisions or dressings, dietary needs or restrictions, and when to make a follow-up appointment. *Comments:*	☐	☐	☐	
10. Have the client or family provide return demonstration of skills required for self-care at home. *Comments:*	☐	☐	☐	
11. Check that transportation to home is available. Check the client's room for any personal belongings. *Comments:*	☐	☐	☐	
12. Complete any paperwork with client as required by agency policy. *Comments:*	☐	☐	☐	

Procedure 29-41	Able to Perform	Able to Perform with Assistance	Unable to Perform	Initials and Date
13. Escort the client to transportation vehicle. *Comments:*	☐	☐	☐	
For Any Discharge				
14. Notify appropriate personnel according to agency policy that the client left the unit. Arrange for room to be cleaned. *Comments:*	☐	☐	☐	
Evaluation				
1. Client encountered no problems in discharge to another facility. *Comments:*	☐	☐	☐	
2. Client, with the assistance of family, is confident about care at home. *Comments:*	☐	☐	☐	

Checklist for Procedure 29-42   Initiating Strict Isolation Precautions

Name _____ Date _____

School _____

Instructor _____

Course _____

Procedure 29-42 Initiating Strict Isolation Precautions	Able to Perform	Able to Perform with Assistance	Unable to Perform	Initials and Date
Assessment				
1. Review physician's orders for isolation to ensure proper setup. *Comments:*	☐	☐	☐	
2. Assess client's and family's understanding of client's condition and reason for isolation to identify required teaching needed. *Comments:*	☐	☐	☐	
Planning/Expected Outcomes				
1. The room will be set up for the appropriate type of isolation. *Comments:*	☐	☐	☐	
2. The client and family will understand the client's condition and the reason for isolation. *Comments:*	☐	☐	☐	
Implementation				
1. Check client's identification band and explain procedure before beginning. Barrier protection must be on before checking the client's identification band. Review physician orders and agency protocols relative to the type of isolation protocols: • Implement protocol related to the type of disinfectant needed to eliminate specific microorganisms. • Alert housekeeping of room number and type of isolation supplies needed in the room. • Make sure the room has the proper ventilation and the bed and other electrical equipment are functioning properly. *Comments:*	☐	☐	☐	
2. Place appropriate isolation supplies outside the client's room and place isolation sign on the door. *Comments:*	☐	☐	☐	

continued on the following page

continued from the previous page

Procedure 29-42	Able to Perform	Able to Perform with Assistance	Unable to Perform	Initials and Date
3. Gather appropriate supplies to take in the room: • Linen • Impermeable bags • Disposable vital signs equipment • Wound care supplies *Comments:*	☐	☐	☐	
4. Remove jewelry, lab coat, and other items not necessary for providing client care. *Comments:*	☐	☐	☐	
5. Wash hands and don disposable clothing: • Apply mask and pinch the metal strip to fit snugly. • Apply cap to cover hair and ears completely, if policy requires a cap. • Apply gown to cover outer garments completely. • Don nonsterile gloves and pull gloves to cover gown's cuff. • Don goggles or face shield. *Comments:*	☐	☐	☐	
6. Enter client's room with all gathered supplies and medications (if the client is to receive medications). *Comments:*	☐	☐	☐	
7. Assess the client's and family's knowledge of the client's diagnosis and isolation: • Reason isolation initiated • Type of isolation • Duration of isolation • How to apply barrier protection *Comments:*	☐	☐	☐	
8. Perform nursing care to meet the needs of the client. Record assessment data on a piece of paper, avoiding contact with any articles in the client's room. *Comments:*	☐	☐	☐	
9. Dispose of soiled articles in the impermeable bags, which should be labeled correctly according to contents. Soiled reusable equipment is removed from the room; label bag accordingly. *Comments:*	☐	☐	☐	

Procedure 29-42	Able to Perform	Able to Perform with Assistance	Unable to Perform	Initials and Date
10. Double-bag soiled linen according to agency policy in an impermeable bag or in plastic linen bag. *Comments:*	☐	☐	☐	
11. Replenish supplies before leaving the client's room and ask the client if anything is needed. *Comments:*	☐	☐	☐	
12. Before leaving, let the client know when you will return and make sure call light is accessible. *Comments:*	☐	☐	☐	
13. Exiting the isolation room: • Untie gown at the waist. • Remove and dispose of gloves. • Grasp and release the ties of the mask and dispose of it. • Release neck ties of the gown and allow gown to fall forward. Place fingers of dominant hand inside cuff of other hand and pull down over other hand. With gown-covered hand, pull gown over the dominant hand. While gown is still on arm, fold outside of gown together, remove, and dispose of it. • Remove cap by slipping your finger under the cap and removing it from the front to back; dispose of it. *Comments:*	☐	☐	☐	
14. Wash hands. Don nonsterile gloves and remove bags from the client's room. Exit room and close door. Dispose of bags according to agency protocol. Remove gloves and wash hands. *Comments:*	☐	☐	☐	
Evaluation				
1. Appropriate type of isolation was instituted. *Comments:*	☐	☐	☐	
2. Client and family express understanding of the client's condition and the reason for isolation. *Comments:*	☐	☐	☐	

Checklist for Procedure 30-1   Surgical Asepsis: Preparing and Maintaining a Sterile Field

Name _____ Date _____

School _____

Instructor _____

Course _____

Procedure 30-1 Surgical Asepsis: Preparing and Maintaining a Sterile Field	Able to Perform	Able to Perform with Assistance	Unable to Perform	Initials and Date
Assessment				
1. Ensure that all packages are dry and intact. Assess sterility of packages. *Comments:*	☐	☐	☐	
2. Assess local environment for a dry, horizontal, stable area. *Comments:*	☐	☐	☐	
Planning/Expected Outcomes				
1. Sterility of the field and all packages, while being opened, will be maintained. *Comments:*	☐	☐	☐	
2. Sterility of the procedure will be maintained. *Comments:*	☐	☐	☐	
Implementation				
1. Wash hands and check the client's identification band. Gather equipment for the type of procedure: • Select only clean, dry packages marked "sterile," and read listing of content. • Check the package for integrity and expiration date. *Comments:*	☐	☐	☐	
2. Select a clean area in the client's environment to establish the sterile field. *Comments:*	☐	☐	☐	
3. Explain procedure to the client; provide specific instructions if client assistance is required during the procedure. *Comments:*	☐	☐	☐	
4. Inquire about and attend to the client's toileting needs. *Comments:*	☐	☐	☐	

continued on the following page

continued from the previous page

Procedure 30-1	Able to Perform	Able to Perform with Assistance	Unable to Perform	Initials and Date
5. Hospital environment: If procedure is to be performed at the client's bedside, the client should be in a private room or moved to a clean treatment room if available. *Comments:*	☐	☐	☐	
6. Home environment: Secure privacy and remove pets from the room. *Comments:*	☐	☐	☐	
7. Position the client and attend to comfort measures; the client's position should provide easy access to the area and facilitate good body mechanics during the procedure. *Comments:*	☐	☐	☐	
8. Wash hands. *Comments:*	☐	☐	☐	
9. Place sterile package (drape or tray) in the center of the clean, dry work area. *Comments:*	☐	☐	☐	
Drape				
10. Open the wrapper, pulling away from the body first. *Comments:*	☐	☐	☐	
11. Grasp the top edge of drape with fingertips of one hand. *Comments:*	☐	☐	☐	
12. Remove the drape by lifting up and away from all objects while it unfolds; discard the outer wrapper with the other hand. *Comments:*	☐	☐	☐	
13. With the free hand, grasp the other drape corner, keeping it away from all objects. *Comments:*	☐	☐	☐	
14. Lay the drape on the surface, with the drape bottom first touching the surface farthest from you; step back and allow the drape to cover the surface. *Comments:*	☐	☐	☐	
Tray				
15. Remove outer wrapping and place the tray on the work surface so that the top flap of the sterile wrapper opens away from you. *Comments:*	☐	☐	☐	

Procedure 30-1	Able to Perform	Able to Perform with Assistance	Unable to Perform	Initials and Date
16. Reach around the tray, not over it. With thumb and index fingertips grasping the wrapper's top flap, gently pull up and then down to open over the surface. *Comments:*	☐	☐	☐	
17. Repeat the same actions to open the side flaps. *Comments:*	☐	☐	☐	
18. Grasp the corner of the bottom flap with fingertips, step back, and pull flap down. *Comments:*	☐	☐	☐	
Adding Additional Sterile Items to Sterile Field				
19. While facing the sterile field, step back, remove outer wrapper, and grasp the item in nondominant hand so that the top flap opens away from you. *Comments:*	☐	☐	☐	
20. With the dominant hand, open the flaps as previously described. *Comments:*	☐	☐	☐	
21. With your dominant hand, pull the wrapper back and away from the sterile field and place the item onto the field. *Comments:*	☐	☐	☐	
22. When adding additional gauze or dressings to the sterile field, open the package as directed, grasp the top flaps of the wrapper and pull downward, then drop the contents onto the center of the field. *Comments:*	☐	☐	☐	
Adding Solutions to Sterile Field				
23. Read the labels and strengths of all solutions three times before pouring. *Comments:*	☐	☐	☐	
24. Remove the lid from the bottle of solution and invert the lid onto a clean surface. *Comments:*	☐	☐	☐	

continued on the following page

continued from the previous page

Procedure 30-1	Able to Perform	Able to Perform with Assistance	Unable to Perform	Initials and Date
25. Hold the bottle, label facing ceiling, 4–6 inches (10–15 c m) over the container on the sterile field; slowly pour the solution into the container to avoid splashing. Pour from the side of the sterile field. *Comments:*	☐	☐	☐	
26. Replace the lid on the container; label the container with the date and time and initial the container. *Comments:*	☐	☐	☐	
Using Sterile Gloves				
27. Wash hands and perform open gloving. *Comments:*	☐	☐	☐	
28. Continue with procedure, keeping gloved hands above waist level at all times and touching only items on the sterile field. *Comments:*	☐	☐	☐	
29. If using a solution to cleanse a site, use sterile forceps to prevent contamination of gloves; dispose of forceps after use or process instruments according to agency policy. *Comments:*	☐	☐	☐	
30. Post procedure, dispose of all contaminated items in appropriate receptacle. *Comments:*	☐	☐	☐	
31. Remove gloves. *Comments:*	☐	☐	☐	
32. Reposition the client. *Comments:*	☐	☐	☐	
33. Clean the environment and wash hands. *Comments:*	☐	☐	☐	
Evaluation				
1. Sterility of field was maintained. *Comments:*	☐	☐	☐	
2. Sterility of procedure was maintained. *Comments:*	☐	☐	☐	

Checklist for Procedure 30-2 Performing Open Gloving

Name _____ Date _____

School _____

Instructor _____

Course _____

Procedure 30-2 Performing Open Gloving	Able to Perform	Able to Perform with Assistance	Unable to Perform	Initials and Date
Assessment				
1. Assess the glove package. Assess the sterility of the glove. *Comments:*	☐	☐	☐	
2. Assess the local environment. A flat, clear work space is necessary to successfully carry out the procedure. *Comments:*	☐	☐	☐	
3. Assess the correct glove size for proper fit. *Comments:*	☐	☐	☐	
Planning/Expected Outcomes				
1. Sterility of the gloves will be maintained while they are being applied. *Comments:*	☐	☐	☐	
2. Sterility of the procedure will be maintained. *Comments:*	☐	☐	☐	
Implementation				
1. Wash hands. *Comments:*	☐	☐	☐	
2. Remove the outer wrapper from the package; place the inner wrapper onto a clean, dry surface. Open inner wrapper to expose gloves. *Comments:*	☐	☐	☐	
3. Identify right and left hand; glove dominant hand first. *Comments:*	☐	☐	☐	
4. Grasp the 2-inch (5-cm)-wide cuff with the thumb and first two fingers of the nondominant hand, touching only the inside of the cuff. *Comments:*	☐	☐	☐	

continued on the following page

continued from the previous page

Procedure 30-2	Able to Perform	Able to Perform with Assistance	Unable to Perform	Initials and Date
5. Gently pull the glove over the dominant hand, making sure the thumb and fingers fit into the proper spaces of the glove. *Comments:*	☐	☐	☐	
6. With the gloved dominant hand, slip your fingers under the cuff of the other glove, gloved thumb abducted, making sure it does not touch any part on your nondominant hand. *Comments:*	☐	☐	☐	
7. Gently slip the glove onto your nondominant hand, making sure the fingers slip into the proper spaces. *Comments:*	☐	☐	☐	
8. With gloved hands, interlock fingers to fit the gloves onto each finger. *Comments:*	☐	☐	☐	
Removing Gloves				
9. If the gloves are soiled, remove as follows: With your dominant hand, grasp the other glove at the wrist. Avoid touching the skin of your wrist with the fingers of the glove. Pull the glove off, turning it inside out. *Comments:*	☐	☐	☐	
10. Place removed glove in palm of gloved hand. *Comments:*	☐	☐	☐	
11. Place thumb of ungloved hand inside the cuff of the glove, touching only the inside of the glove. *Comments:*	☐	☐	☐	
12. Pull glove off, turning it inside out and over the other glove. *Comments:*	☐	☐	☐	
13. Dispose of soiled gloves according to institutional policy and wash hands. *Comments:*	☐	☐	☐	
Evaluation				
1. Sterility of the gloves, sterile field, and procedure was maintained without breaks. *Comments:*	☐	☐	☐	

Checklist for Procedure 30-3   Performing Urinary Catheterization: Female/Male

Name _____ Date _____

School _____

Instructor _____

Course _____

Procedure 30-3 **Performing Urinary Catheterization: Female/Male**	**Able to Perform**	**Able to Perform with Assistance**	**Unable to Perform**	**Initials and Date**
Assessment				
1. Assess the need for catheterization and the type of catheterization ordered. Use latex-free catheter if client has latex allergy. *Comments:*	☐	☐	☐	
2. Assess for the need for perineal care before catheterization. *Comments:*	☐	☐	☐	
3. Assess the urinary meatus for signs of infection or inflammation. Ask the client for any history of difficulty with prior catheterizations, anxiety, or urinary strictures. *Comments:*	☐	☐	☐	
4. Assess the client's ability to assist with the procedure. *Comments:*	☐	☐	☐	
5. Assess the light. *Comments:*	☐	☐	☐	
6. Assess for an allergy to povidone-iodine and/or latex. *Comments:*	☐	☐	☐	
7. Watch for indications of distress or embarrassment. Explore further if indicated. *Comments:*	☐	☐	☐	
Planning/Expected Outcomes				
1. The catheter will be inserted without pain, trauma, or injury to the client. *Comments:*	☐	☐	☐	
2. The client's bladder will be emptied without complication. *Comments:*	☐	☐	☐	

continued on the following page

continued from the previous page

Procedure 30-3	Able to Perform	Able to Perform with Assistance	Unable to Perform	Initials and Date
3. The nurse will maintain the sterility of the catheter during insertion. *Comments:*	☐	☐	☐	
Implementation				
1. Explain procedure before beginning. Gather the equipment needed. *Comments:*	☐	☐	☐	
2. Identify client by reading arm band. Assess two client identifiers. *Comments:*	☐	☐	☐	
3. Provide for privacy. Assess for allergy to povidone-iodine. *Comments:*	☐	☐	☐	
4. Set the bed to a comfortable height to work and raise the opposite side rail. *Comments:*	☐	☐	☐	
5. Assist the client to a supine position with legs spread and feet together. *Comments:*	☐	☐	☐	
6. Drape the client's abdomen and thighs for warmth if needed. *Comments:*	☐	☐	☐	
7. Ensure adequate lighting of the perineal area. *Comments:*	☐	☐	☐	
8. Wash hands; apply disposable gloves. *Comments:*	☐	☐	☐	
9. Wash perineal area. *Comments:*	☐	☐	☐	
10. Remove gloves and wash hands. *Comments:*	☐	☐	☐	

Procedure 30-3	Able to Perform	Able to Perform with Assistance	Unable to Perform	Initials and Date
11. Remove plastic wrap from catheterization kit. Place catheterization kit between client's legs and open the catheterization kit, using aseptic technique. • Open the top flap away from your body by grasping the corner of the outer surface between your thumb and finger only. • Grasp the outer surface of the left and right flaps and open. • Grasp the proximal (closest) flap and open toward your body. Avoid touching the inside of the flap with your hands or clothing. *Comments:*	☐	☐	☐	
12. Add the catheter or any other items needed using sterile technique. *Comments:*	☐	☐	☐	
13. Apply sterile gloves. *Comments:*	☐	☐	☐	
14. Place the sterile drape from the catheterization kit between the client's thighs, close to the perineum, being careful not to touch nonsterile areas with sterile gloves. *Comments:*	☐	☐	☐	
15. If inserting a retention catheter, attach the syringe filled with sterile water to the Luer-lock tail of the catheter. Inflate and deflate the retention balloon. *Comments:*	☐	☐	☐	
16. Keep water-filled syringe attached to the port. Attach the catheter to the urine drainage bag. *Comments:*	☐	☐	☐	
17. Open supplies: • Open povidone-iodine or other antimicrobial solution and pour over cotton balls. • Squeeze lubrication package onto sterile field. *Comments:*	☐	☐	☐	
18. Coat the distal portion of the catheter with water-soluble, sterile lubricant and place it nearby on sterile field. *Comments:*	☐	☐	☐	

continued on the following page

continued from the previous page

Procedure 30-3	Able to Perform	Able to Perform with Assistance	Unable to Perform	Initials and Date
Performing Female Urinary Catheterization				
19. Place the fenestrated drape over the client's perineal area with the labia visible through the opening. *Comments:*	☐	☐	☐	
20. Gently spread the labia minora with the fingers of your nondominant hand and visualize the urinary meatus. *Comments:*	☐	☐	☐	
21. Holding the labia apart with your nondominant hand, use the forceps to pick up a cotton ball soaked in povidone-iodine and cleanse the periurethral mucosa. Use one downward stroke for each cotton ball and dispose. Keep the labia separated with your nondominant hand until you insert the catheter. *Comments:*	☐	☐	☐	
22. Holding the catheter in the dominant hand, steadily insert the catheter into the meatus until urine is noted in the drainage bag or tubing. *Comments:*	☐	☐	☐	
23. If the catheter will be removed as soon as the client's bladder is empty, insert the catheter another inch and hold the catheter in place as the bladder drains. *Comments:*	☐	☐	☐	
24. If the catheter will be indwelling with a retention balloon, continue inserting another 1–3 inches. *Comments:*	☐	☐	☐	
25. Inflate the retention balloon using the manufacturer's recommendations or according to the health care provider's instructions. *Comments:*	☐	☐	☐	
26. Instruct the client to immediately report discomfort or pressure during balloon inflation; if pain occurs, discontinue the procedure, deflate the balloon, and insert the catheter farther into the urethra. If the client continues to complain of pain with balloon inflation, remove the catheter and notify the client's health care provider. *Comments:*	☐	☐	☐	

Procedure 30-3	Able to Perform	Able to Perform with Assistance	Unable to Perform	Initials and Date
27. Once the balloon has been inflated, gently pull the catheter until the retention balloon is resting snug against the bladder neck. *Comments:*	☐	☐	☐	
28. Secure the catheter according to institutional policy. Securing the catheter to the client's thigh is usually acceptable; be sure to leave enough slack so that it does not pull on the bladder. *Comments:*	☐	☐	☐	
29. Place the drainage bag below the level of the bladder. Do not let it rest on the floor. Make sure the tubing lies over, not under, the leg. *Comments:*	☐	☐	☐	
30. Wash the perineal area with soap and water. *Comments:*	☐	☐	☐	
31. Dispose of equipment, remove gloves, and wash hands. *Comments:*	☐	☐	☐	
32. Assist client to a comfortable position and lower the bed. *Comments:*	☐	☐	☐	
33. Assess the color, odor, quality, and amount of urine. *Comments:*	☐	☐	☐	
34. Wash hands. *Comments:*	☐	☐	☐	
Performing Male Urinary Catheterization				
35. Repeat Actions 1–14. *Comments:*	☐	☐	☐	
36. Place the fenestrated drape over the client's perineal area with the penis extending through the opening. *Comments:*	☐	☐	☐	

continued on the following page

continued from the previous page

Procedure 30-3	Able to Perform	Able to Perform with Assistance	Unable to Perform	Initials and Date
37. If inserting a retention catheter, attach the syringe filled with sterile water to the Luer-lock tail of the catheter. Inflate and deflate the retention balloon. Keep water-filled syringe attached to the port. *Comments:*	☐	☐	☐	
38. Attach the catheter to the urine drainage bag if it is not preconnected. *Comments:*	☐	☐	☐	
39. Open povidone-iodine or other antimicrobial solution and pour over cotton balls. Remove the cap from the water-soluble lubricant syringe. *Comments:*	☐	☐	☐	
40. With your nondominant hand, gently grasp the penis and retract the foreskin (if present). With your dominant hand, use the forceps to pick up a saturated cotton ball. Place the cotton ball on the meatus. Using a circular motion, cleanse from the meatus to the base of the penis. Discard cotton ball. Cleanse the meatus three times using a new saturated cotton ball each time. *Comments:*	☐	☐	☐	
41. Hold the penis perpendicular to the body and pull up gently. *Comments:*	☐	☐	☐	
42. Inject 10 mL sterile, water-soluble lubricant into the urethra. *Comments:*	☐	☐	☐	
43. Holding the catheter in the dominant hand, steadily insert the catheter about 8 inches, until urine is noted in the drainage bag or tubing. *Comments:*	☐	☐	☐	
44. If the catheter will be removed as soon as the client's bladder is empty, insert the catheter another inch, place the penis in a comfortable position, and hold the catheter in place as the bladder drains. *Comments:*	☐	☐	☐	
45. If the catheter will be indwelling with a retention balloon, continue inserting until the hub of the catheter is met. *Comments:*	☐	☐	☐	

Procedure 30-3	Able to Perform	Able to Perform with Assistance	Unable to Perform	Initials and Date
46. Inflate the retention balloon with sterile water per manufacturer's recommendations or according to the health care provider's orders. *Comments:*	☐	☐	☐	
47. If the client experiences pain during balloon inflation, deflate the balloon and insert the catheter farther into the bladder. If the pain continues with balloon inflation, remove the catheter and notify the client's health care provider. *Comments:*	☐	☐	☐	
48. Once the balloon has been inflated, gently pull the catheter until the retention balloon is resting snugly against the bladder neck. *Comments:*	☐	☐	☐	
49. Secure the catheter to the client's thigh according to institutional policy. Allow enough slack in the catheter so it will not pull on the bladder. *Comments:*	☐	☐	☐	
50. Place the drainage bag below the level of the bladder. Do not let it rest on the floor. Make sure the tubing lies over, not under, the legs. *Comments:*	☐	☐	☐	
51. Clean perineal area with soap and water, and dry the area. *Comments:*	☐	☐	☐	
52. Dispose of equipment, remove gloves, and wash hands. *Comments:*	☐	☐	☐	
53. Assist the client to a comfortable position. Lower the bed. *Comments:*	☐	☐	☐	
54. Assess and document the amount, color, odor, and quality of urine. *Comments:*	☐	☐	☐	
55. Wash hands. *Comments:*	☐	☐	☐	

continued from the previous page

Procedure 30-3	Able to Perform	Able to Perform with Assistance	Unable to Perform	Initials and Date
Evaluation				
1. Catheter was inserting without pain, trauma, or injury to the client. *Comments:*	☐	☐	☐	
2. Client's bladder was emptied without complication. *Comments:*	☐	☐	☐	
3. Nurse maintained the sterility of the catheter during insertion. *Comments:*	☐	☐	☐	

Checklist for Procedure 30-4　Irrigating a Urinary Catheter

Name _____ Date _____

School _____

Instructor _____

Course _____

Procedure 30-4 **Irrigating a Urinary Catheter**	**Able to Perform**	**Able to Perform with Assistance**	**Unable to Perform**	**Initials and Date**
Assessment				
1. Assess the written order for type of irrigation, purpose of the irrigation, type and amount of solution to irrigate with, any premedication ordered, and any other details of the order. *Comments:*	☐	☐	☐	
2. Assess the condition of the client as it relates to the procedure: patency of the catheter, characteristics of urinary drainage, and total intake and output status of the client. *Comments:*	☐	☐	☐	
3. Assess for current pain or bladder spasms. *Comments:*	☐	☐	☐	
4. Assess the client's knowledge about the procedure. *Comments:*	☐	☐	☐	
5. If this is a repeat of the procedure, read the charting from previous nurses. *Comments:*	☐	☐	☐	
Planning/Expected Outcomes				
1. The urinary catheter will be patent. *Comments:*	☐	☐	☐	
2. Sediment/blood clots will be passed through the catheter. *Comments:*	☐	☐	☐	
3. The bladder will be free of sources of local irritation. *Comments:*	☐	☐	☐	
4. The urinary pH will be assisted to a more acidic state. *Comments:*	☐	☐	☐	

continued on the following page

continued from the previous page

Procedure 30-4	Able to Perform	Able to Perform with Assistance	Unable to Perform	Initials and Date
Implementation				
1. Check client's identification band and explain procedure before beginning. Verify the need for bladder or catheter irrigation. *Comments:*	☐	☐	☐	
2. For prn catheter irrigation, palpate for full bladder and check current output against previous totals. *Comments:*	☐	☐	☐	
3. Check health care provider's orders for type of irrigation, irrigant, and the amount. *Comments:*	☐	☐	☐	
4. If this is a repeat procedure, read previous documentation in the record. *Comments:*	☐	☐	☐	
5. Assemble all supplies. *Comments:*	☐	☐	☐	
6. Premedicate client if ordered or needed. *Comments:*	☐	☐	☐	
7. Educate client as needed, based on what the client already knows. *Comments:*	☐	☐	☐	
8. Provide for client privacy with a closed door or curtain. *Comments:*	☐	☐	☐	
9. Assist the client to a dorsal recumbent position. *Comments:*	☐	☐	☐	
10. Wash hands. *Comments:*	☐	☐	☐	
11. Apply clean gloves and empty the collection bag of urine. *Comments:*	☐	☐	☐	

Procedure 30-4	Able to Perform	Able to Perform with Assistance	Unable to Perform	Initials and Date
12. Remove gloves and wash hands. *Comments:*	☐	☐	☐	
13. Expose the indwelling catheter and place the water-resistant drape underneath it. *Comments:*	☐	☐	☐	
14. Open the sterile syringe and container. Stand it up carefully in or on the wrapper and add 100–200 mL sterile diluent without touching or contaminating the tip of the syringe or the inside of the receptacle. *Comments:*	☐	☐	☐	
15. Open the antiseptic swab package, exposing the swab sticks and the sterile cover for drainage tube. *Comments:*	☐	☐	☐	
16. Apply the sterile gloves. *Comments:*	☐	☐	☐	
17. Using the antiseptic swab sticks, disinfect the connection between the catheter and the drainage tubing. *Comments:*	☐	☐	☐	
18. After disinfectant dries, loosen the ends of the connection. *Comments:*	☐	☐	☐	
19. Grasp the catheter and tubing 1–2 inches from their ends, with the catheter in the nondominant hand. *Comments:*	☐	☐	☐	
20. Fold the catheter to pinch the catheter closed between the palm and last three fingers; use the thumb and first finger to hold the sterile cap for the drainage tube. *Comments:*	☐	☐	☐	
21. Separate the catheter and tube, covering the tube tightly with the sterile cap. *Comments:*	☐	☐	☐	

continued on the following page

continued from the previous page

Procedure 30-4	Able to Perform	Able to Perform with Assistance	Unable to Perform	Initials and Date
22. Fill the syringe: 30 mL for catheter irrigation, 60 mL for bladder irrigation. Insert the tip of the syringe into the catheter and gently instill the solution into the catheter. *Comments:*	☐	☐	☐	
23. Clamp catheter if ordered. If not clamped, irrigant may be released into a collection container or aspirated back into the syringe. *Comments:*	☐	☐	☐	
24. If the bladder or catheter is being irrigated to clear solid material, repeat irrigation until return is clear. *Comments:*	☐	☐	☐	
25. Reconnect system and remove sterile gloves. Wash hands. *Comments:*	☐	☐	☐	
26. Record the type of irrigation, total amount of irrigant used, and the color and quality of return. *Comments:*	☐	☐	☐	
27. Monitor client for pain, urine color and clarity, any solid material passed, and total intake and output. *Comments:*	☐	☐	☐	
28. Wash hands. *Comments:*	☐	☐	☐	
Evaluation				
1. Urinary catheter remains patent. *Comments:*	☐	☐	☐	
2. Any sediment/blood clots were passed through the catheter. *Comments:*	☐	☐	☐	
3. Bladder is free of local irritation. *Comments:*	☐	☐	☐	
4. Urinary pH was more acidic. *Comments:*	☐	☐	☐	

Checklist for Procedure 30-5   Irrigating the Bladder Using a Closed-System Catheter

Name _____ Date _____

School _____

Instructor _____

Course _____

Procedure 30-5 **Irrigating the Bladder Using a** **Closed-System Catheter**	**Able to Perform**	**Able to Perform with Assistance**	**Unable to Perform**	**Initials and Date**
Assessment				
1. Assess the client for bladder distension or complaints of fullness or discomfort. *Comments:*	☐	☐	☐	
2. Assess the drainage system for equal or larger amounts of drainage versus infused irrigant. *Comments:*	☐	☐	☐	
3. Assess the color, consistency, and clarity of the bladder drainage, noting any clots or debris present. *Comments:*	☐	☐	☐	
Planning/Expected Outcomes				
1. The client will not exhibit signs or symptoms of bladder or urinary tract infection. *Comments:*	☐	☐	☐	
2. The client will not experience pain or discomfort. *Comments:*	☐	☐	☐	
3. The catheter will remain patent, and the bladder will not be distended. *Comments:*	☐	☐	☐	
Implementation				
Intermittent Bladder Irrigation Using a Standard Indwelling Catheter and a Y Adapter				
1. Check client's identification band and explain procedure before beginning. Wash hands. *Comments:*	☐	☐	☐	
2. Close privacy curtain or door. *Comments:*	☐	☐	☐	
3. Hang the prescribed irrigation solution from an IV pole. *Comments:*	☐	☐	☐	

continued on the following page

continued from the previous page

Procedure 30-5	Able to Perform	Able to Perform with Assistance	Unable to Perform	Initials and Date
4. Insert the clamped irrigation tubing into the bottle of irrigant and prime the tubing with fluid, expel all air, and reclamp the tube. *Comments:*	☐	☐	☐	
5. Prepare sterile antiseptic swabs and sterile Y connector if one was used. *Comments:*	☐	☐	☐	
6. Clamp the urinary catheter. *Comments:*	☐	☐	☐	
7. Apply sterile gloves. *Comments:*	☐	☐	☐	
8. Unhook the drainage bag from the indwelling catheter. *Comments:*	☐	☐	☐	
9. While holding the drainage tubing and the drainage port of the catheter in your nondominant hand, cleanse both the drainage tubing and the drainage port with antiseptic swabs. *Comments:*	☐	☐	☐	
10. Connect one port of the Y connector to the drainage port of the catheter. *Comments:*	☐	☐	☐	
11. Connect another port of the Y adapter to the drainage tubing. *Comments:*	☐	☐	☐	
12. Attach the third port of the Y adapter to the irrigant tubing. *Comments:*	☐	☐	☐	
13. Unclamp the urinary catheter and establish the urine is draining through the catheter into the drainage bag. *Comments:*	☐	☐	☐	
14. To irrigate the catheter and bladder, clamp the drainage tubing distal to the Y adapter. *Comments:*	☐	☐	☐	

Procedure 30-5	Able to Perform	Able to Perform with Assistance	Unable to Perform	Initials and Date
15. Unclamp irrigation tubing and instill the prescribed amount of irrigant. *Comments:*	☐	☐	☐	
16. Clamp the irrigant tubing. *Comments:*	☐	☐	☐	
17. If the irrigant is to remain in the bladder for a measured length of time, wait the prescribed length of time. *Comments:*	☐	☐	☐	
18. Unclamp the drainage tubing and monitor the drainage as it flows into the drainage bag. *Comments:*	☐	☐	☐	
Closed Bladder Irrigation Using a Three-Way Catheter				
19. Follow Actions 1–4. *Comments:*	☐	☐	☐	
20. Prepare sterile antiseptic swabs and any other sterile equipment needed. *Comments:*	☐	☐	☐	
21. Clamp the urinary catheter. *Comments:*	☐	☐	☐	
22. Apply sterile gloves. *Comments:*	☐	☐	☐	
23. Remove the cap from the irrigation port of the three-way catheter. *Comments:*	☐	☐	☐	
24. Cleanse the irrigation port with the sterile antiseptic swabs. *Comments:*	☐	☐	☐	
25. Attach the irrigation tubing to the irrigation port of the three-way catheter. *Comments:*	☐	☐	☐	

continued on the following page

continued from the previous page

Procedure 30-5	Able to Perform	Able to Perform with Assistance	Unable to Perform	Initials and Date
26. Remove the clamp from the catheter and observe for urine drainage. *Comments:*	☐	☐	☐	
27. **If intermittent irrigation has been ordered:** Follow Actions 15–16. *Comments:*	☐	☐	☐	
28. If the irrigant is to remain in the bladder for a measured time, clamp the drainage tube before instilling the irrigant and wait the prescribed length of time. *Comments:*	☐	☐	☐	
29. Monitor the drainage as it flows into the drainage bag. *Comments:*	☐	☐	☐	
30. **If continuous bladder irrigation has been ordered:** Adjust the clamp on the irrigation tubing to allow the prescribed rate of irrigant to flow into the catheter and bladder. *Comments:*	☐	☐	☐	
31. Monitor the drainage for color, clarity, debris, and volume as it flows back into the drainage bag. *Comments:*	☐	☐	☐	
32. Tape the catheter securely to the thigh. *Comments:*	☐	☐	☐	
33. Remove gloves and wash hands. *Comments:*	☐	☐	☐	
Evaluation				
1. Client does not exhibit signs or symptoms of bladder or urinary tract infection. *Comments:*	☐	☐	☐	
2. Client has not experienced pain or discomfort as a result of the bladder irrigation. *Comments:*	☐	☐	☐	
3. Catheter remains patent, and the client's bladder is not distended. *Comments:*	☐	☐	☐	

Checklist for Procedure 30-6   Changing a Bowel Diversion Ostomy Appliance: Pouching a Stoma

Name _____ Date _____

School _____

Instructor _____

Course _____

Procedure 30-6 Changing a Bowel Diversion Ostomy Appliance: Pouching a Stoma	Able to Perform	Able to Perform with Assistance	Unable to Perform	Initials and Date
Assessment				
1. Inspect the stoma for color and texture. Comments:	☐	☐	☐	
2. Inspect the condition of the skin surrounding the stoma. Comments:	☐	☐	☐	
3. Measure the dimensions of the stoma before obtaining ostomy appliance system from a central supply. Comments:	☐	☐	☐	
Planning/Expected Outcomes				
1. The peristomal skin integrity will remain intact. Comments:	☐	☐	☐	
2. Irritated or denuded peristomal skin will heal. Comments:	☐	☐	☐	
3. The client will acknowledge the change in body image. Comments:	☐	☐	☐	
4. The client will express positive feelings about self. Comments:	☐	☐	☐	
5. The client will maintain fluid balance. Comments:	☐	☐	☐	
Implementation				
1. Check client's identification band and explain procedure before beginning. Wash hands. Comments:	☐	☐	☐	
2. Assemble drainable pouch and wafer. Comments:	☐	☐	☐	

continued on the following page

continued from the previous page

Procedure 30-6	Able to Perform	Able to Perform with Assistance	Unable to Perform	Initials and Date
3. Apply clean gloves. *Comments:*	☐	☐	☐	
4. Remove current ostomy appliance after emptying pouch of stool, if present. *Comments:*	☐	☐	☐	
5. Dispose of appliance in appropriate waste container. *Comments:*	☐	☐	☐	
6. Remove gloves and wash hands. *Comments:*	☐	☐	☐	
7. Apply clean gloves. *Comments:*	☐	☐	☐	
8. Cleanse stoma and skin with warm tap water. Pat dry. *Comments:*	☐	☐	☐	
9. Measure stoma using a measuring guide for appropriate length and width of stoma at base. *Comments:*	☐	☐	☐	
10. Place gauze pad over orifice of stoma to wick stool while preparing the wafer and pouch for application. *Comments:*	☐	☐	☐	
11. Trace pattern onto paper backing of wafer. *Comments:*	☐	☐	☐	
12. Cut wafer as traced. *Comments:*	☐	☐	☐	
13. Attach clean pouch to wafer. Make sure port closure is closed. *Comments:*	☐	☐	☐	
14. Remove gauze pad from orifice of stoma. *Comments:*	☐	☐	☐	
15. Remove paper backing from wafer and place on skin with stoma centered in cutout opening of wafer. *Comments:*	☐	☐	☐	

Procedure 30-6	Able to Perform	Able to Perform with Assistance	Unable to Perform	Initials and Date
16. Tape the wafer edges down with hypoallergenic tape (optional). *Comments:*	☐	☐	☐	
17. Dispose of used materials, remove gloves and wash hands. *Comments:*	☐	☐	☐	
Evaluation				
1. Peristomal skin integrity remains intact. *Comments:*	☐	☐	☐	
2. Irritated or denuded peristomal skin integrity is healed. *Comments:*	☐	☐	☐	
3. Client acknowledges the change in body image. *Comments:*	☐	☐	☐	
4. Client expresses positive feelings about self. *Comments:*	☐	☐	☐	
5. Client maintains fluid balance. *Comments:*	☐	☐	☐	

Checklist for Procedure 30-7   Application of Heat and Cold

Name _____ Date _____

School _____

Instructor _____

Course _____

Procedure 30-7 Application of Heat and Cold	Able to Perform	Able to Perform with Assistance	Unable to Perform	Initials and Date
Assessment				
1. Assess the area to receive heat or cold treatment for circulation. *Comments:*	☐	☐	☐	
2. Assess the skin sensation and integrity around the area to be treated. *Comments:*	☐	☐	☐	
3. Assess for open wounds that may be affected by the treatment. *Comments:*	☐	☐	☐	
4. Check the client's systemic temperature. *Comments:*	☐	☐	☐	
5. Assess age. *Comments:*	☐	☐	☐	
Planning/Expected Outcomes				
1. The client will derive the intended benefits of the heat or cold treatment. *Comments:*	☐	☐	☐	
2. The client will not experience any injury to skin integrity. *Comments:*	☐	☐	☐	
Implementation				
Moist Heat				
1. Check client's identification band and explain procedure before beginning. Check the health care provider's order and reason for the warm compress. *Comments:*	☐	☐	☐	
2. Wash hands. *Comments:*	☐	☐	☐	

continued on the following page

continued from the previous page

Procedure 30-7	Able to Perform	Able to Perform with Assistance	Unable to Perform	Initials and Date
3. Assess the client's skin for areas of redness, breakdown, or scar tissue. If open wounds are involved, carefully assess the open wounds. Explain to client the reason for the compress. *Comments:*	☐	☐	☐	
4. Review the client's condition, medical diagnosis, and any history of diabetes mellitus or impairments in sensation. *Comments:*	☐	☐	☐	
5. Warm the container of sterile saline or tap water by placing it in a bath basin filled with hot tap water. Sterile saline should be warmed to 105°–113°F. If you are using a commercial compress, follow the manufacturer's directions for heating it. *Comments:*	☐	☐	☐	
6. Place a waterproof pad under the body area that needs the warm compress. *Comments:*	☐	☐	☐	
7. Pour the sterile saline into the sterile basin. Soak an appropriate-size piece of gauze or a towel, wring out the excess saline, and place it on the affected area. Wear gloves if there is any drainage of the client's body fluids. Wear sterile gloves if there is an open wound. *Comments:*	☐	☐	☐	
8. Wrap the area with a waterproof pad or apply disposable heat or aquathermia pad. *Comments:*	☐	☐	☐	
9. Check the client's skin periodically for signs of heat intolerance. Tell the client to report any signs of discomfort immediately. *Comments:*	☐	☐	☐	
10. If tolerated, leave the compress in place for approximately 20 minutes and then remove it. *Comments:*	☐	☐	☐	
11. Dry the affected area with sterile towels if there is an open wound and with clean towels if there is no open wound. *Comments:*	☐	☐	☐	

Procedure 30-7	Able to Perform	Able to Perform with Assistance	Unable to Perform	Initials and Date
12. Properly dispose of all single-use equipment according to hospital protocol. *Comments:*	☐	☐	☐	
13. Remove gloves and wash hands. *Comments:*	☐	☐	☐	
14. Reassess the condition of the client's skin. *Comments:*	☐	☐	☐	
15. Record the procedure: condition of the client's skin and length of time of moist heat application. Report any abnormal findings to the physician. *Comments:*	☐	☐	☐	
Sitz Bath				
16. Wash hands and assemble equipment. *Comments:*	☐	☐	☐	
17. Run tap water to preferred temperature (between 100° and 110° F). Have the client test the temperature on the dorsal surface of the wrist. *Comments:*	☐	☐	☐	
18. For toilet-insert model, raise the seat of the toilet. Set the basin on the rim of the toilet bowl. Fill water bag and prime tubing. Close the clamp. Hang water bag above the toilet. Thread tubing through the front of the basin. Secure the tubing in the notch in the bottom of the basin. *Comments:*	☐	☐	☐	
19. For stand-alone model, fill basin with water. *Comments:*	☐	☐	☐	
20. Pad seat with a towel. *Comments:*	☐	☐	☐	
21. Always use Standard Precautions when assisting with perineal care treatments. Have client remove and dispose of peri-pad in a biohazard receptacle. *Comments:*	☐	☐	☐	

continued on the following page

continued from the previous page

Procedure 30-7	Able to Perform	Able to Perform with Assistance	Unable to Perform	Initials and Date
22. Ensure that the floor is dry. Assist the client to bathroom, if necessary. *Comments:*	☐	☐	☐	
23. Have the client sit in the basin. For the toilet-insert model, demonstrate how to unclamp the tubing to start the water flow. *Comments:*	☐	☐	☐	
24. Cover the client's lap for warmth and modesty. *Comments:*	☐	☐	☐	
25. Ensure that the client can reach the call button. Instruct the client to call before standing up. *Comments:*	☐	☐	☐	
26. After 20 minutes, help the client dry the area by gently patting with clean towels. *Comments:*	☐	☐	☐	
27. Assist the client to bed. Encourage the client to lie flat or elevate hips for 20 minutes. *Comments:*	☐	☐	☐	
28. For toilet-insert model, empty remaining water into toilet. Rinse basin and bag. Clean according to institutional policy. For stand-alone model, empty water from drain trap into basin. Clean according to institutional policy. *Comments:*	☐	☐	☐	
Dry Heat				
29. Check the order and the purpose of the heat treatment. *Comments:*	☐	☐	☐	
30. Determine whether there are any underlying problems that may affect the use of heat treatment, such as decreased sensation; decreased mentation; or a history of diabetes mellitus, bleeding disorders, peripheral vascular disease, or peripheral neuropathy. Heat should not be used over areas of scarring. *Comments:*	☐	☐	☐	

Procedure 30-7	Able to Perform	Able to Perform with Assistance	Unable to Perform	Initials and Date
31. Wash hands. *Comments:*	☐	☐	☐	
32. Check the skin for lotions or ointments and remove if present. *Comments:*	☐	☐	☐	
33. Gather equipment and complete as follows: For a disposable heat pack: • Activate the pack according to the manufacturer's directions. • Wrap the pack in a towel or protective covering. Do not use pins. Use tape if needed to secure the towel. • Discard after use. For an Aquathermia pad: • Follow manufacturer's directions. • Fill the control unit with distilled water or as indicated by manufacturer's directions. • Check the control unit and tubing for leaks. Turn on the unit and check the temperature of the water with a thermometer (proper temperature, 105° F). *Comments:*	☐	☐	☐	
34. Wash hands. *Comments:*	☐	☐	☐	
Application of Cold				
35. Wash hands. *Comments:*	☐	☐	☐	
36. Assess the client's sensation and skin color at the site of planned application. Determine if any tissue damage is present. Assess for bleeding or wound drainage. *Comments:*	☐	☐	☐	
37. Identify whether the client has a history of circulatory impairment or neuropathy. *Comments:*	☐	☐	☐	
38. Check the order and the reason for the application of cold. *Comments:*	☐	☐	☐	

continued on the following page

continued from the previous page

Procedure 30-7	Able to Perform	Able to Perform with Assistance	Unable to Perform	Initials and Date
39. If using ice bag with moist gauze or towels, fill the bag three-fourths full with ice and remove the air from the bag. Close the bag. Check for leaks. Wrap the bag in a towel or protective cover and place on the affected area. If cold soaks are being applied, use the appropriate-size basin for the body part to be soaked. *Comments:*	☐	☐	☐	
40. If using an ice collar: Fill the collar three-fourths full with ice and remove the air from the collar before closing the collar. Check for leaks. Place the collar in a protective cover and around the client's neck. *Comments:*	☐	☐	☐	
41. If a disposable cold pack is used, activate the pack according to the manufacturer's directions, wrap the pack in a towel, and place it on the affected area. Some packs come with covers. Secure pack in place with tape, elastic wrap, or bandage. Dispose of the pack after the treatment. *Comments:*	☐	☐	☐	
42. Assess the client's skin periodically for signs of cold intolerance or tissue damage. *Comments:*	☐	☐	☐	
43. If the client can tolerate the cold, leave the cold application in place for approximately 20 minutes at approximately 15°C (59°F). *Comments:*	☐	☐	☐	
44. Dispose of equipment according to agency policy. *Comments:*	☐	☐	☐	
45. Reassess the condition of the client's skin or exposed tissue. *Comments:*	☐	☐	☐	
46. Wash hands. *Comments:*	☐	☐	☐	
Evaluation				
1. Client derived intended benefits of the heat or cold treatment. *Comments:*	☐	☐	☐	
2. Client had no injury to skin integrity. *Comments:*	☐	☐	☐	

Checklist for Procedure 30-8   Administering Oral, Sublingual, and Buccal Medications

Name _____ Date _____

School _____

Instructor _____

Course _____

Procedure 30-8 Administering Oral, Sublingual, and Buccal Medications	Able to Perform	Able to Perform with Assistance	Unable to Perform	Initials and Date
Assessment				
1. Assess the seven rights: right client, right medication, right route, right dose, right time, right to refuse, and right documentation. *Comments:*	☐	☐	☐	
2. Review the action, purpose, normal dosage and route, common side effects, time of onset and peak action, and nursing implications of each drug. *Comments:*	☐	☐	☐	
3. Assess the client's condition to be sure the order of the health care provider is appropriate. *Comments:*	☐	☐	☐	
4. Assess the client's ability to swallow food and fluid. *Comments:*	☐	☐	☐	
5. Assess for any contraindications for oral medication, such as nausea and vomiting, gastric suction, or gastric surgery resulting in decreased peristalsis. *Comments:*	☐	☐	☐	
6. Assess the client's medical record for allergies to food or medications. *Comments:*	☐	☐	☐	
7. Assess the client's knowledge about the use of medications. *Comments:*	☐	☐	☐	
8. Assess the client's age. *Comments:*	☐	☐	☐	
9. Assess the client's need for fluids. *Comments:*	☐	☐	☐	

continued on the following page

continued from the previous page

Procedure 30-8	Able to Perform	Able to Perform with Assistance	Unable to Perform	Initials and Date
10. Assess the client's ability to sit or turn to the side. *Comments:*	☐	☐	☐	
Planning/Expected Outcomes				
1. The client will swallow the prescribed medication. *Comments:*	☐	☐	☐	
2. The client will be able to explain the medication's purpose and schedule for taking medication. *Comments:*	☐	☐	☐	
3. The client will have no gastrointestinal discomfort or alterations in function. *Comments:*	☐	☐	☐	
4. The client will show the desired response to the medication. *Comments:*	☐	☐	☐	
5. The client will not have an allergic reaction. *Comments:*	☐	☐	☐	
Implementation				
1. Wash hands. *Comments:*	☐	☐	☐	
2. Arrange the medication tray and cups; follow institutional protocol. *Comments:*	☐	☐	☐	
3. Unlock the medication cart or log on to the computer. *Comments:*	☐	☐	☐	
4. Prepare medication for one client at a time following the seven rights. Select the correct drug from the medication drawer according to the MAR. Calculate the drug dosage if needed. *Comments:*	☐	☐	☐	

Procedure 30-8	Able to Perform	Able to Perform with Assistance	Unable to Perform	Initials and Date
5. To prepare a tablet or capsule: • Select the correct drug from the medication drawer according to the MAR. Calculate the drug dosage if needed. Pour tablets into the medication cup without touching them. • Scored tablets may be broken, if necessary, using gloved hands or with a pill-cutting device. • A unit dose tablet should be placed directly into the medicine cup without opening it until it is administered to the client. • For clients with difficulty swallowing, some tablets may be crushed into a powder using a mortar and pestle or by being placed between two paper medication cups and ground with a blunt object. *Time released and specially coated medications must not be crushed.* Comments:	☐	☐	☐	
6. To prepare a liquid medication: • Remove the bottle cap and place cap upside down. • Hold the bottle with the label up and place the medication cup at eye level on a level surface while pouring. • Fill the cup to the desired level using the surface or base of the meniscus as the scale, not the edge of the liquid on the cup. • Wipe the bottle with a paper towel. Comments:	☐	☐	☐	
7. To prepare a narcotic, obtain the key to the narcotic drawer and check the narcotic record for the drug count when signing out the dose. If the drug count does not agree with the record, report to charge nurse immediately. Comments:	☐	☐	☐	
8. Check expiration date on all medications. • Double-check the medication administration record (MAR) with the prepared drugs and place with the client's medications. • Return stock medications to their shelf or drawer. • Do not leave drugs unattended. Comments:	☐	☐	☐	

continued from the previous page

Procedure 30-8	Able to Perform	Able to Perform with Assistance	Unable to Perform	Initials and Date
9. Administer medications to the client: • Observe the correct time to give the medication. • Identify the client using two identifiers by reading the client's name bracelet, repeating the name, and/or asking the client to state his or her name. Additionally, check the hospital number if name alert or client is not reliable. • Check the drug packaging if it is present to ensure the medication type and dosage. • Assess the client's condition and the form of the medication. • Perform any assessment required for specific medications, such as a pulse or blood pressure. • Explain the purpose of the drug and answer any questions, assessing the client's sixth right to refuse the medication. • Assist the client to a sitting or lateral position. • Allow the client to hold the tablet or medication cup. • Give a glass of liquid, and straw if needed. • For *sublingual* medications, instruct the client to dissolve medication under the tongue and allow it to dissolve completely. • For *buccal* medications, instruct the client to dissolve medication in the mouth against the cheek. • For medications given through a *nasogastric tube,* crush tablets or open capsules and dissolve with 20–30 mL of warm water in a cup. Be sure medication will still be properly absorbed if crushed and dissolved. Check placement of the feeding tube or nasogastric tube before instilling anything but air into the tube. • Remain with the client until each medication has been swallowed or dissolved. • Assist the client into a comfortable position. *Comments:*	☐	☐	☐	
10. Dispose of soiled supplies and wash hands. *Comments:*	☐	☐	☐	
11. Document (seventh right) the time and route of medication administration on the MAR and return it to the client's file. *Comments:*	☐	☐	☐	
12. Return the cart; clean and restock as needed. Clean work area. *Comments:*	☐	☐	☐	

Procedure 30-8	Able to Perform	Able to Perform with Assistance	Unable to Perform	Initials and Date
Evaluation				
1. Evaluate client's response to the drug within 30 minutes of administration or sooner if an allergic reaction is anticipated. *Comments:*	☐	☐	☐	
2. Ask client or caregiver to discuss the purpose, action, dosage schedule, and side effects of the drug. *Comments:*	☐	☐	☐	

Checklist for Procedure 30-9   Withdrawing Medication from an Ampule

Name _____ Date _____

School _____

Instructor _____

Course _____

Procedure 30-9 **Withdrawing Medication from an Ampule**	Able to Perform	Able to Perform with Assistance	Unable to Perform	Initials and Date
Assessment				
1. Identify the correct ampule, including medication, dosage strength, dosage volume, dosage route, and expiration date, to avoid medication error. *Comments:*	☐	☐	☐	
2. Assess the syringe, filter needle, and injection needle for expiration date and package intactness to evaluate the sterility of the equipment. *Comments:*	☐	☐	☐	
3. Assess the fluid in the ampule for cloudiness, particulate matter, or color changes. *Comments:*	☐	☐	☐	
4. Identify the medication's intended action, purpose, normal dosage range, time of action, common side effects, and nursing implications. *Comments:*	☐	☐	☐	
Planning/Expected Outcomes				
1. The correct medication ampule will be selected. *Comments:*	☐	☐	☐	
2. The medication will be drawn into an appropriate syringe. *Comments:*	☐	☐	☐	
3. Microorganisms will not be introduced into the sterile system. *Comments:*	☐	☐	☐	
4. Foreign objects will not be introduced into the sterile system. *Comments:*	☐	☐	☐	

continued on the following page

continued from the previous page

Procedure 30-9	Able to Perform	Able to Perform with Assistance	Unable to Perform	Initials and Date
Implementation				
1. Wash hands. *Comments:*	☐	☐	☐	
2. Select appropriate ampule. *Comments:*	☐	☐	☐	
3. Select syringe with filter needle. *Comments:*	☐	☐	☐	
4. Obtain a sterile gauze pad. *Comments:*	☐	☐	☐	
5. Select and set aside the appropriate length of safety needle for planned injection. *Comments:*	☐	☐	☐	
6. Clear a work space. *Comments:*	☐	☐	☐	
7. Observe ampule for location of the medication. *Comments:*	☐	☐	☐	
8. If medication is trapped in the top, flick the neck of the ampule repeatedly with your fingernail while holding the ampule upright. *Comments:*	☐	☐	☐	
9. Wrap the sterile gauze pad around the neck and snap off the top in an outward motion directed away from self. *Comments:*	☐	☐	☐	
10. Invert ampule, place the needle into the liquid. Gently withdraw medication fluid into the syringe. *Comments:*	☐	☐	☐	
11. Alternately, place the ampule on the counter, hold, and tilt slightly with the nondominant hand. Insert the needle below the level of liquid and gently draw liquid into the syringe, tilting the ampule as needed to reach all the liquid. *Comments:*	☐	☐	☐	

Procedure 30-9	Able to Perform	Able to Perform with Assistance	Unable to Perform	Initials and Date
12. Remove the filter needle and replace with the safety injection needle. *Comments:*	☐	☐	☐	
13. Dispose of filter needle and glass ampule in appropriate sharps container. *Comments:*	☐	☐	☐	
14. Label the syringe with drug, dose, date, and time. *Comments:*	☐	☐	☐	
15. Wash hands. *Comments:*	☐	☐	☐	
Evaluation				
1. Correct medication ampule was selected. *Comments:*	☐	☐	☐	
2. Medication was drawn into an appropriate syringe. *Comments:*	☐	☐	☐	
3. Microorganisms were not introduced into the sterile system. *Comments:*	☐	☐	☐	
4. Foreign objects were not introduced into the sterile system. *Comments:*	☐	☐	☐	

Checklist for Procedure 30-10   Withdrawing Medication from a Vial

Name _____ Date _____

School _____

Instructor _____

Course _____

Procedure 30-10 Withdrawing Medication from a Vial	Able to Perform	Able to Perform with Assistance	Unable to Perform	Initials and Date
Assessment				
1. Assess the expiration date on the vial to be sure it is current. Comments:	☐	☐	☐	
2. Assess the contents of the vial for the correct medication and dosage. Comments:	☐	☐	☐	
3. Assess the contents of the vial for color, consistency, and debris. Comments:	☐	☐	☐	
4. Assess the integrity of the vial and the stopper. Comments:	☐	☐	☐	
5. Assess the integrity of the syringe and needle that will be used to withdraw the medication. Comments:	☐	☐	☐	
Planning/Expected Outcomes				
1. The correct medication will be drawn from the vial using sterile technique. Comments:	☐	☐	☐	
2. The correct dose will be drawn from the vial. Comments:	☐	☐	☐	
3. The remaining contents of multiuse vials will not be contaminated. Comments:	☐	☐	☐	
4. The date the vial was opened will be marked on the vial in ink. Comments:	☐	☐	☐	

continued on the following page

continued from the previous page

Procedure 30-10	Able to Perform	Able to Perform with Assistance	Unable to Perform	Initials and Date
Implementation				
1. Wash hands. Apply gloves. *Comments:*	☐	☐	☐	
2. Select the appropriate vial. *Comments:*	☐	☐	☐	
3. Verify health care provider's orders. *Comments:*	☐	☐	☐	
4. Check expiration date on vial. *Comments:*	☐	☐	☐	
5. Determine the medication route and select the appropriate-size syringe and needle. *Comments:*	☐	☐	☐	
6. While holding the syringe at eye level, withdraw the plunger to the desired volume of medication. *Comments:*	☐	☐	☐	
7. Clean the rubber top of the vial with a 70% alcohol pad. Use a circular motion, starting at the center and working out. *Comments:*	☐	☐	☐	
8. Using sterile technique, uncap the needle and lay the needle cap on a clean surface. *Comments:*	☐	☐	☐	
9. Placing the needle in the center of the vial, inject air slowly. Do not cause turbulence. *Comments:*	☐	☐	☐	
10. Invert the vial and slowly, using gentle negative pressure, withdraw the medication. Keep the needle tip in the medication. *Comments:*	☐	☐	☐	
11. With the syringe at eye level, determine that the appropriate dose/volume has been reached. *Comments:*	☐	☐	☐	

Procedure 30-10	Able to Perform	Able to Perform with Assistance	Unable to Perform	Initials and Date
12. Slowly withdraw the needle from the vial. Follow the institution's policy regarding recapping and changing needles. *Comments:*	☐	☐	☐	
13. Using ink, mark the current date, time, and initials on the vial. *Comments:*	☐	☐	☐	
14. Label the syringe with drug, the dose, date, and time. *Comments:*	☐	☐	☐	
15. Wash hands. *Comments:*	☐	☐	☐	
Evaluation				
1. The vial was current and the rubber seal intact. *Comments:*	☐	☐	☐	
2. The correct amount of medication was withdrawn. *Comments:*	☐	☐	☐	
3. The needle did not become contaminated or damaged. *Comments:*	☐	☐	☐	

Checklist for Procedure 30-11   Administering an Intradermal Injection

Name _____ Date _____

School _____

Instructor _____

Course _____

Procedure 30-11 Administering an Intradermal Injection	Able to Perform	Able to Perform with Assistance	Unable to Perform	Initials and Date
Assessment				
1. Assess the seven rights: right client, right medication, right route, right dose, right time, right to refuse, and right documentation. Comments:	☐	☐	☐	
2. Review health care provider's order. Comments:	☐	☐	☐	
3. Review information regarding the expected reaction to the allergen. Comments:	☐	☐	☐	
4. Assess for the indications for intradermal injection, including the client's allergy history. Comments:	☐	☐	☐	
5. Check the expiration date of the medication vial. Comments:	☐	☐	☐	
6. Assess the client's knowledge regarding the medication to be received. Comments:	☐	☐	☐	
7. Assess the client's response to discussion about an injection. Comments:	☐	☐	☐	
Planning/Expected Outcomes				
1. The client will experience minimal pain or burning at the injection site. Comments:	☐	☐	☐	
2. The client will experience no allergic reaction or side effects from the injection. Comments:	☐	☐	☐	

continued on the following page

continued from the previous page

Procedure 30-11	Able to Perform	Able to Perform with Assistance	Unable to Perform	Initials and Date
3. The client will be able to explain the significance of the presence or absence of a skin reaction. *Comments:*	☐	☐	☐	
4. The client will keep follow-up appointments within the recommended time frame to have responses to the medication evaluated. *Comments:*	☐	☐	☐	
Implementation				
1. Check client's identification band and explain procedure before beginning. Wash hands and put on clean gloves. *Comments:*	☐	☐	☐	
2. Provide privacy. Identify client, and assess right to refuse (sixth right). *Comments:*	☐	☐	☐	
3. Select injection site. • Inspect skin for bruises, inflammation, edema, masses, tenderness, and sites of previous injections. • Forearm site should be three to four finger widths below antecubital space and one hand width above wrists on inner aspect of forearm. *Comments:*	☐	☐	☐	
4. Select 1-mL tuberculin syringe and one-quarter- to five-eighths-inch 25- to 27-gauge needle. *Comments:*	☐	☐	☐	
5. Assist the client into a comfortable position. • Relax the arm, with forearm extended on a flat surface. • Distract the client by talking about an interesting subject. *Comments:*	☐	☐	☐	
6. Use alcohol pad antiseptic swab in a circular motion to clean skin at site. *Comments:*	☐	☐	☐	
7. Pull cap from needle. *Comments:*	☐	☐	☐	

Procedure 30-11	Able to Perform	Able to Perform with Assistance	Unable to Perform	Initials and Date
8. Administer injection: • With nondominant hand, stretch skin over site with forefinger and thumb. • Insert needle slowly at a 5- to 15-degree angle, bevel up, until resistance is felt; then advance no more than one-eighth of an inch below the skin. The needle tip should be seen through the skin. • Slowly inject the medication. Resistance will be felt. • Note a small blob forming under the skin surface. *Comments:*	☐	☐	☐	
9. Withdraw the needle, applying gentle pressure with the antiseptic swab. *Comments:*	☐	☐	☐	
10. Do not massage the site. *Comments:*	☐	☐	☐	
11. Assist the client to a comfortable position. *Comments:*	☐	☐	☐	
12. Discard the uncapped needle and syringe in a sharps container. *Comments:*	☐	☐	☐	
13. Remove gloves and wash hands. *Comments:*	☐	☐	☐	

Evaluation

	Able to Perform	Able to Perform with Assistance	Unable to Perform	Initials and Date
1. Client experienced only minimal pain or burning at the injection site. *Comments:*	☐	☐	☐	
2. Client experienced no allergic reaction or other side effects from the injection. *Comments:*	☐	☐	☐	
3. Client was able to explain the significance of the presence or absence of a skin reaction. *Comments:*	☐	☐	☐	

continued on the following page

continued from the previous page

Procedure 30-11	**Able to Perform**	**Able to Perform with Assistance**	**Unable to Perform**	**Initials and Date**
4. Client kept all follow-up appointments within the recommended time frame to have responded to the medication evaluated. *Comments:*	☐	☐	☐	

Checklist for Procedure 30-12   Administering a Subcutaneous Injection

Name _____ Date _____

School _____

Instructor _____

Course _____

Procedure 30-12 **Administering a Subcutaneous Injection**	Able to Perform	Able to Perform with Assistance	Unable to Perform	Initials and Date
Assessment				
1. Assess the seven rights: right client, right medication, right route, right dose, right time, right to refuse, and right documentation. *Comments:*	☐	☐	☐	
2. Review health care provider's order. *Comments:*	☐	☐	☐	
3. Review information regarding the drug ordered, such as action, purpose, normal dosage and route, common side effects, time of onset and peak action, and nursing implications. *Comments:*	☐	☐	☐	
4. Assess client for factors that may influence an injection, such as circulatory shock or reduced local tissue perfusion. *Comments:*	☐	☐	☐	
5. Assess for previous subcutaneous injections. *Comments:*	☐	☐	☐	
6. Assess for the indications for subcutaneous injection. *Comments:*	☐	☐	☐	
7. Assess the client's age. *Comments:*	☐	☐	☐	
8. Assess the client's knowledge regarding the medication. *Comments:*	☐	☐	☐	
9. Assess the client's response to discussion about an injection. *Comments:*	☐	☐	☐	

continued on the following page

continued from the previous page

Procedure 30-12	Able to Perform	Able to Perform with Assistance	Unable to Perform	Initials and Date
10. Check the client's drug allergy history as an allergic reaction could occur. *Comments:*	☐	☐	☐	
Planning/Expected Outcomes				
1. The client will experience minimal pain or burning at the injection site. *Comments:*	☐	☐	☐	
2. The client will experience no allergic reaction or other side effects from the injection. *Comments:*	☐	☐	☐	
3. The client will be able to explain the action, side effects, dosage, and schedule of the medication, and rationale for rotation of sites. *Comments:*	☐	☐	☐	
Implementation				
1. Check client's identification band and explain procedure prior to beginning. Wash hands and put on clean gloves. *Comments:*	☐	☐	☐	
2. Provide privacy. Identify client using two different identifiers. *Comments:*	☐	☐	☐	
3. Select injection site. • Inspect skin for bruises, inflammation, edema, masses, tenderness, and sites of previous injections and avoid these areas. • Use subcutaneous tissue around the abdomen, lateral aspects of upper arm or thigh, or scapular area. *Comments:*	☐	☐	☐	
4. Select needle size. • Measure skinfold by grasping skin between thumb and forefinger. • Be sure needle is one-half the length of the skinfold from top to bottom. *Comments:*	☐	☐	☐	

Procedure 30-12	Able to Perform	Able to Perform with Assistance	Unable to Perform	Initials and Date
5. Assist the client into a comfortable position. • Relax the arm, leg, or abdomen. • Distract the client by talking about an interesting subject or explaining what you are doing step by step. *Comments:*	☐	☐	☐	
6. Use alcohol pad antiseptic swab to clean skin at site. *Comments:*	☐	☐	☐	
7. While holding swab between fingers, pull cap from needle. *Comments:*	☐	☐	☐	
8. Administer injection: • Hold syringe between thumb and forefinger of dominant hand like a dart. • Pinch skin with nondominant hand. • Inject needle quickly and firmly (like a dart) at a 45-degree to 90-degree angle. • Release the skin. • Grasp the lower end of the syringe with nondominant hand and position dominant hand at the end of the plunger. Do not move the syringe. • Pull back on the plunger to ascertain that the needle is not in a vein. If no blood appears, slowly inject the medication. (Aspiration is contraindicated with some medications; check with the pharmacy if you are unclear.) *Comments:*	☐	☐	☐	
9. Withdraw the needle while applying pressure with the swab. Do not push down on the needle with swab while withdrawing it, because this will cause more pain. *Comments:*	☐	☐	☐	
10. Apply pressure. Some medications should not be massaged. Ask the pharmacy if you are unclear. *Comments:*	☐	☐	☐	
11. Discard the uncapped needle and syringe appropriately. *Comments:*	☐	☐	☐	
12. Assist the client to a comfortable position. *Comments:*	☐	☐	☐	

continued on the following page

continued from the previous page

Procedure 30-12	Able to Perform	Able to Perform with Assistance	Unable to Perform	Initials and Date
13. Remove gloves and wash hands. *Comments:*	☐	☐	☐	
Evaluation				
1. Client experienced only minimal pain or burning at the injection site. *Comments:*	☐	☐	☐	
2. Assessed client's response to the medication 30 minutes after administration. *Comments:*	☐	☐	☐	
3. Asked client to discuss the purpose, action, dosage schedule, and side effects of the medication. *Comments:*	☐	☐	☐	

Checklist for Procedure 30-13   Administering an Intramuscular Injection

Name _____ Date _____

School _____

Instructor _____

Course _____

Procedure 30-13 Administering an Intramuscular Injection	Able to Perform	Able to Perform with Assistance	Unable to Perform	Initials and Date
Assessment				
1. Assess the seven rights: right client, right medication, right route, right dose, right time, right to refuse, and right documentation. *Comments:*	☐	☐	☐	
2. Review health care provider's order. *Comments:*	☐	☐	☐	
3. Review information regarding the drug ordered, such as action, purpose, normal dosage and route, common side effects, time of onset and peak action, and nursing implications. *Comments:*	☐	☐	☐	
4. Assess the client for factors that may influence an injection, such as circulatory shock, reduced local tissue perfusion, or muscle atrophy. *Comments:*	☐	☐	☐	
5. Assess for previous intramuscular injections. *Comments:*	☐	☐	☐	
6. Assess for the indications for intramuscular injections. *Comments:*	☐	☐	☐	
7. Assess the client's age. *Comments:*	☐	☐	☐	
8. Assess the client's knowledge regarding the medication to be received. *Comments:*	☐	☐	☐	
9. Assess the client's response to discussion about an injection. *Comments:*	☐	☐	☐	

continued on the following page

continued from the previous page

Procedure 30-13	Able to Perform	Able to Perform with Assistance	Unable to Perform	Initials and Date
10. Assess the client's size and muscle development. *Comments:*	☐	☐	☐	
11. Check the client's allergy history. *Comments:*	☐	☐	☐	
Planning/Expected Outcomes				
1. The correct client will receive the correct medication. *Comments:*	☐	☐	☐	
2. The client will experience only minimal pain or burning at the injection site. *Comments:*	☐	☐	☐	
3. The client will experience no allergic reaction or other side effects from the injection. *Comments:*	☐	☐	☐	
4. The client will be able to explain the action, side effects, dosage, and schedule of the medication. *Comments:*	☐	☐	☐	
5. The client will obtain the expected benefit from the medication. *Comments:*	☐	☐	☐	
6. The client will not experience pain or skin staining secondary to the medication when Z-track injection is given. *Comments:*	☐	☐	☐	
Implementation				
1. Check client's identification band and explain procedure before beginning. Wash hands and put on clean gloves. *Comments:*	☐	☐	☐	
2. Provide privacy. Identify client using two different identifiers. *Comments:*	☐	☐	☐	
3. Select injection site. • Inspect skin for bruises, inflammation, edema, masses, tenderness, and sites of previous injections. • Use anatomic landmarks. *Comments:*	☐	☐	☐	

Procedure 30-13	Able to Perform	Able to Perform with Assistance	Unable to Perform	Initials and Date
4. Select needle size. Assess size and weight of client and site to be used. *Comments:*	☐	☐	☐	
5. Assist the client into a comfortable position. • Vastus lateralis—lying flat or supine with knee slightly flexed. • Ventrogluteal—lying on side or back with knee and hip slightly flexed. • Dorsogluteal—lying prone with feet turned inward or on side with upper knee and hip flexed and placed in front of lower leg. • Deltoid—standing with arm relaxed at side or sitting with lower arm relaxed on lap or lying flat with lower arm relaxed across abdomen. • Distract the client by talking about an interesting subject. *Comments:*	☐	☐	☐	
6. Use antiseptic swab to clean skin at site. *Comments:*	☐	☐	☐	
7. While holding swab between fingers of nondominant hand, pull cap from needle. *Comments:*	☐	☐	☐	
8. Administer injection: • Hold syringe between thumb and forefinger of dominant hand like a dart. • Spread skin tightly or pinch a generous section of tissue firmly—for cachetic clients. • Inject needle quickly and firmly (like a dart) at a 90-degree angle. • Release the skin. • Grasp the lower end of the syringe with nondominant hand and position dominant hand at the end of the plunger. Do not move the syringe. • Pull back on the plunger and aspirate to ascertain if needle is in a vein. If no blood appears, inject the medication. *Comments:*	☐	☐	☐	
9. Remove nondominant hand and quickly withdraw the needle while applying pressure with the antiseptic swab. *Comments:*	☐	☐	☐	

continued on the following page

continued from the previous page

Procedure 30-13	Able to Perform	Able to Perform with Assistance	Unable to Perform	Initials and Date
10. Apply pressure. Certain protocols suggest gentle massage action. *Comments:*	☐	☐	☐	
11. Discard the uncapped needle and syringe in a specified biohazard sharps container. *Comments:*	☐	☐	☐	
12. Assist the client to a comfortable position. *Comments:*	☐	☐	☐	
13. Remove gloves and wash hands. *Comments:*	☐	☐	☐	
Z-Track Injection				
14. Create an airlock. Add 0.1–0.2 ml of air to the dose in the syringe. The air will push the medication out of the needle when the last of the medication has been injected. *Comments:*	☐	☐	☐	
15. Wash hands and put on gloves. *Comments:*	☐	☐	☐	
16. Use an antiseptic swab to clean skin at site. *Comments:*	☐	☐	☐	
17. Pull the skin and subcutaneous tissue to the side or downward about an inch, out of alignment with the underlying muscle. (Do not use this technique in the deltoid; dorsogluteal is the preferred site.) *Comments:*	☐	☐	☐	
18. Using sterile technique, remove the needle guard with your nondominant hand. *Comments:*	☐	☐	☐	
19. While maintaining traction on the skin, using your dominant hand, dart the needle into the skin at a 90-degree angle. *Comments:*	☐	☐	☐	

Procedure 30-13	Able to Perform	Able to Perform with Assistance	Unable to Perform	Initials and Date
20. Aspirate for a minimum of 5 seconds. Observe for blood return. *Comments:*	☐	☐	☐	
21. If no blood return present, slowly (at a rate of 1mL/10 seconds) inject the medication. *Comments:*	☐	☐	☐	
22. Allow the needle to stay in place for 10 seconds after the injection. *Comments:*	☐	☐	☐	
23. While maintaining traction on the skin, remove the needle and allow the skin to return to its normal position. *Comments:*	☐	☐	☐	
24. Do not rub or wipe the skin after removal of the needle. *Comments:*	☐	☐	☐	
25. Discard the uncapped needle and syringe appropriately. *Comments:*	☐	☐	☐	
26. Assist the client to a comfortable position. *Comments:*	☐	☐	☐	
27. Remove gloves and wash hands. *Comments:*	☐	☐	☐	
Evaluation				
1. Correct client received the correct medication. *Comments:*	☐	☐	☐	
2. Client experienced only minimal pain, burning, numbness, or tingling at the injection site. *Comments:*	☐	☐	☐	
3. Assess the client's response to medication 10–30 minutes later. *Comments:*	☐	☐	☐	

continued on the following page

continued from the previous page

Procedure 30-13	Able to Perform	Able to Perform with Assistance	Unable to Perform	Initials and Date
4. Client is able to discuss the purpose, action, schedule, and side effects of the medication. *Comments:*	☐	☐	☐	
5. Client obtained the expected benefit. *Comments:*	☐	☐	☐	

Checklist for Procedure 30-14   Administering Eye and Ear Medications

Name _____ Date _____

School _____

Instructor _____

Course _____

Procedure 30-14 **Administering Eye and Ear Medications**	Able to Perform	Able to Perform with Assistance	Unable to Perform	Initials and Date
Assessment				
1. Assess the seven rights: right client, right medication, right route, right dose, right time, right to refuse, and right documentation. *Comments:*	☐	☐	☐	
2. Assess the condition of the client's eyes and/or ears. *Comments:*	☐	☐	☐	
3. Assess the medication order. *Comments:*	☐	☐	☐	
Planning/Expected Outcomes				
1. The correct client will receive the medication according to the seven rights. *Comments:*	☐	☐	☐	
2. The client will encounter the minimum of discomfort during the medication administration procedure. *Comments:*	☐	☐	☐	
3. The client will receive maximum benefit from the medication. *Comments:*	☐	☐	☐	
Implementation				
Eye Medication 1. Check client's identification band and explain procedure before beginning. Check for allergies or other contraindications. *Comments:*	☐	☐	☐	
2. Gather the necessary equipment. *Comments:*	☐	☐	☐	
3. Follow the seven rights of drug administration. *Comments:*	☐	☐	☐	

continued on the following page

continued from the previous page

Procedure 30-14	Able to Perform	Able to Perform with Assistance	Unable to Perform	Initials and Date
4. Take the medication to the client's room and place on a clean surface. *Comments:*	☐	☐	☐	
5. Check the client's identification band. *Comments:*	☐	☐	☐	
6. Assist the client as needed if client wants to instill medication. *Comments:*	☐	☐	☐	
7. Wash hands. Apply nonsterile latex-free gloves if needed. *Comments:*	☐	☐	☐	
8. Place the client in a supine position with the head slightly hyperextended. *Comments:*	☐	☐	☐	
Instilling Eyedrops				
9. Remove cap from bottle and place cap on its side. *Comments:*	☐	☐	☐	
10. Place a tissue below the lower lid. *Comments:*	☐	☐	☐	
11. With nondominant hand, hold eyedropper one-half to three-fourths inch above the eyeball; rest hand on client's forehead to stabilize. *Comments:*	☐	☐	☐	
12. Place hand on cheekbone and expose lower conjunctival sac by pulling down on cheek. *Comments:*	☐	☐	☐	
13. While the client looks up, drop prescribed number of drops into center of conjunctival sac. *Comments:*	☐	☐	☐	
14. While the client closes and moves eyes, place fingers on either side of the client's nose to close the tear ducts and prevent the medication from draining out of the eye. *Comments:*	☐	☐	☐	

Procedure 30-14	Able to Perform	Able to Perform with Assistance	Unable to Perform	Initials and Date
15. Remove gloves and wash hands. *Comments:*	☐	☐	☐	
16. Document (seventh right) on the MAR the route, site (which eye), and the time administered. *Comments:*	☐	☐	☐	
Eye Ointment Application				
17. Repeat Actions 3 and 5–8. *Comments:*	☐	☐	☐	
Lower Lid				
18. • With nondominant hand, gently separate the client's eyelids with thumb and forefinger and grasp lower lid near margin immediately below the lashes; exert downward pressure over the cheek. • Instruct the client to look up. • Apply eye ointment along inside edge of the entire lower eyelid, from inner to outer canthus. *Comments:*	☐	☐	☐	
Upper Lid				
19. • Instruct the client to look down. • With nondominant hand, gently grasp lashes near center of upper lid with thumb and index finger and draw lid up and away from eyeball. • Squeeze ointment along upper lid starting at inner canthus. *Comments:*	☐	☐	☐	
20. Repeat Actions 15 and 16. *Comments:*	☐	☐	☐	
Medication Disk				
21. Repeat Actions 1–8. *Comments:*	☐	☐	☐	
22. Open package and press dominant, sterile gloved finger against the disk so that it lies lengthwise across fingertips. *Comments:*	☐	☐	☐	
23. Instruct the client to look up. *Comments:*	☐	☐	☐	

continued on the following page

continued from the previous page

Procedure 30-14	Able to Perform	Able to Perform with Assistance	Unable to Perform	Initials and Date
24. With nondominant hand, gently pull the client's lower eyelid down and place the disk horizontally in the conjunctival sac. • Pull the lower eyelid out, up, and over the disk. • Instruct the client to blink several times. • If disk is still visible, repeat steps. • Once disk is in place, instruct the client to gently press the fingers against the closed lids; do not rub eyes or move the disk across the cornea. • If the disk falls out, rinse it under cool water and reinsert. *Comments:*	☐	☐	☐	
25. If the disk is prescribed for both eyes, repeat Actions 22–24. *Comments:*	☐	☐	☐	
26. Repeat Actions 14–16. *Comments:*	☐	☐	☐	
Removing an Eye Medication Disk				
27. Repeat Actions 3 and 5–8. *Comments:*	☐	☐	☐	
28. Remove the disk: • With nondominant hand, invert the lower eyelid and identify the disk. • If the disk is located in the upper eye, instruct the client to close the eye, and place your finger on the closed eyelid. Apply gentle, long, circular strokes; instruct the client to open the eye. Disk should be located in corner of eye. With your fingertip, slide the disk to the lower lid, then proceed. • With dominant hand, use the forefinger to slide the disk onto the lid and out of the client's eye. *Comments:*	☐	☐	☐	
29. Remove gloves and wash hands. *Comments:*	☐	☐	☐	
30. Record on the MAR the removal of the disk. *Comments:*	☐	☐	☐	
Ear Medication				
1. Check with the client and chart for any known allergies. *Comments:*	☐	☐	☐	
2. Check the MAR against the health care provider's written orders. *Comments:*	☐	☐	☐	

Procedure 30-14	Able to Perform	Able to Perform with Assistance	Unable to Perform	Initials and Date
3. Wash hands. *Comments:*	☐	☐	☐	
4. Place the client in a side-lying position with the affected ear facing up. *Comments:*	☐	☐	☐	
5. Straighten the ear canal by pulling the pinna down and back for children younger than 3 years or upward and outward in adults and older children. *Comments:*	☐	☐	☐	
6. Instill the drops into the ear canal; hold dropper one-half inch above ear canal. *Comments:*	☐	☐	☐	
7. Ask the client to maintain the position for 2–3 minutes. *Comments:*	☐	☐	☐	
8. Place a cotton ball on the outermost part of the canal. *Comments:*	☐	☐	☐	
9. Wash hands. *Comments:*	☐	☐	☐	
Evaluation				
1. Correct client received the right dose of the medication via the right route at the right time. *Comments:*	☐	☐	☐	
2. Procedure was performed with minimum trauma and/or discomfort to the client. *Comments:*	☐	☐	☐	
3. Client received maximum benefit from the medication. *Comments:*	☐	☐	☐	
4. All prescribed medication went into the eye or ear, and none was spilled. *Comments:*	☐	☐	☐	

Checklist for Procedure 30-15   Administering Skin/Topical Medications

Name _____ Date _____

School _____

Instructor _____

Course _____

Procedure 30-15 Administering Skin/Topical Medications	Able to Perform	Able to Perform with Assistance	Unable to Perform	Initials and Date
Assessment				
1. Assess the seven rights: right client, right medication, right route, right dose, right time, right to refuse, and right documentation. *Comments:*	☐	☐	☐	
2. Assess the the area where treatment will be applied. *Comments:*	☐	☐	☐	
3. If drug is for systemic effect, assess for area free of scars, moles, or other skin aberrations. *Comments:*	☐	☐	☐	
4. Check the client's allergy history. *Comments:*	☐	☐	☐	
Planning/Expected Outcomes				
1. The client's skin integrity will be maintained. *Comments:*	☐	☐	☐	
2. The client will experience relief of itching, irritation, or pain. *Comments:*	☐	☐	☐	
3. The client will experience the maximum effect from the medication. *Comments:*	☐	☐	☐	
Implementation				
1. Check client's identification band and explain procedure before beginning. Wash hands. *Comments:*	☐	☐	☐	
2. Obtain order for medication from health care provider. *Comments:*	☐	☐	☐	

continued on the following page

continued from the previous page

Procedure 30-15	Able to Perform	Able to Perform with Assistance	Unable to Perform	Initials and Date
3. Ascertain the client's allergic status. *Comments:*	☐	☐	☐	
4. If unfamiliar with medication, read label and insert, or seek appropriate information. *Comments:*	☐	☐	☐	
5. Select medication and verify medication with orders (first medication verification). *Comments:*	☐	☐	☐	
6. Check medication expiration date. *Comments:*	☐	☐	☐	
7. Read medication label again before leaving medication room or cart as available in facilities (second medication verification). *Comments:*	☐	☐	☐	
8. Take the medication to the client's room and introduce self. In some facilities, topical medications used for skin irritations are kept in the client's room, so verification must be done at the bedside. *Comments:*	☐	☐	☐	
9. Ask the client if he or she has had the medication before and to describe its effect. Ascertain client's allergy status. *Comments:*	☐	☐	☐	
10. Explain the purpose of the medication. *Comments:*	☐	☐	☐	
11. Read the label for the third time (third medication verification) and check the client's identification band. *Comments:*	☐	☐	☐	
12. Position the client appropriately for administration of medication. Provide privacy. *Comments:*	☐	☐	☐	

Procedure 30-15	Able to Perform	Able to Perform with Assistance	Unable to Perform	Initials and Date
13. Put on gloves. If dressing is over area to be treated, remove, discard, and change gloves. *Comments:*	☐	☐	☐	
14. Clean the skin surface thoroughly and pat skin dry. • Open wound: clean area to be treated with mild soap and water. • Irritated skin: use only warm water. • Systemically absorbed topical medication: clean skin surface thoroughly and pat skin dry, leaving no residues of soap. • Do not rub vigorously because absorption can be altered. *Comments:*	☐	☐	☐	
15. Assess the client's skin condition, making notation of circulation, drainage, color, temperature, or any altered skin integrity. *Comments:*	☐	☐	☐	
16. Change gloves. *Comments:*	☐	☐	☐	
17. Apply medication according to label. If lotion or ointment, apply a thin layer and smooth into skin as indicated. *Comments:*	☐	☐	☐	
18. If an aerosol spray is used, shake the container and administer according to directions. Spray evenly over affected area, and avoid spraying close to client's or caregiver's face. *Comments:*	☐	☐	☐	
19. If gels or pastes are used, applicators may be needed. Apply evenly. If applying over an area with hair growth, follow direction of hair. *Comments:*	☐	☐	☐	
20. If powders are used, dust lightly and avoid inhalation by client and caregiver. *Comments:*	☐	☐	☐	

continued on the following page

continued from the previous page

Procedure 30-15	Able to Perform	Able to Perform with Assistance	Unable to Perform	Initials and Date
21. If nitroglycerin ointment or paste is used: • Remove the old ointment strip and clean the old site. New ointment will be applied in a different area. • Cleanse the new site with the appropriate cleaner. • Squeeze the dose out onto the enclosed measuring strip before applying it to the client. • Flatten the roll of ointment to spread it over a wider area. • Apply the measuring paper, ointment side down, to a nonhairy portion of the client's body. • Tape the paper in place. *Comments:*	☐	☐	☐	
22. If a transdermal patch is used: • Follow the manufacturer's directions and apply the patch to a smooth cleaned skin surface. • Remove the old patch and wash the site of the old patch. • Wash and prepare the skin at a new site. • Remove the protective covering and apply the new patch. *Comments:*	☐	☐	☐	
23. Write the date and time on the patch. Remove gloves and wash hands. *Comments:*	☐	☐	☐	
24. Document (seventh right) the medication given, the site it was applied to, and the client's response to the mediation. *Comments:*	☐	☐	☐	
Evaluation				
1. Client's skin integrity was maintained. *Comments:*	☐	☐	☐	
2. Client experienced relief of itching, irritation, or pain if this was the intent of the medication. *Comments:*	☐	☐	☐	
3. Client experienced maximum effect from the topical medication. *Comments:*	☐	☐	☐	
4. Client experienced no allergic reaction. *Comments:*	☐	☐	☐	

Checklist for Procedure 30-16   Administering Nasal Medications

Name _____ Date _____

School _____

Instructor _____

Course _____

Procedure 30-16 Administering Nasal Medications	Able to Perform	Able to Perform with Assistance	Unable to Perform	Initials and Date
Assessment				
1. Assess the seven rights: right client, right medication, right route, right dose, right time, right to refuse, and right documentation. *Comments:*	☐	☐	☐	
2. Assess the client's nasal congestion and nasal obstruction. *Comments:*	☐	☐	☐	
3. Assess the color, quantity, and odor of the client's discharge and the color and moistness of the nasal mucosa. *Comments:*	☐	☐	☐	
4. Assess the client's pain and/or discomfort level in the area of the sinuses. *Comments:*	☐	☐	☐	
5. Assess the client for systemic conditions that may be adversely affected by nasal medications. *Comments:*	☐	☐	☐	
Planning/Expected Outcomes				
1. The client will be free of nasal congestion. *Comments:*	☐	☐	☐	
2. The client will be free of nasal discharge and odor. *Comments:*	☐	☐	☐	
3. The client will breathe freely through the nasal passages. *Comments:*	☐	☐	☐	
4. The client will be free of sinus pain and nasal pain. *Comments:*	☐	☐	☐	

continued on the following page

continued from the previous page

Procedure 30-16	Able to Perform	Able to Perform with Assistance	Unable to Perform	Initials and Date
5. The client's nasal passages will be moist and pink. *Comments:*	☐	☐	☐	
Implementation				
1. Check client's identification band and explain procedure before beginning. Wash hands. Wear a mask if the client is coughing or sneezing. Don latex-free gloves. *Comments:*	☐	☐	☐	
2. Explain the purpose of the medication and the position desired for the client. *Comments:*	☐	☐	☐	
3. Explain the sensation of the medications. If drops are used, explain to the client that a sensation of medications may be felt in the posterior oral pharynx. *Comments:*	☐	☐	☐	
4. Have the client clear the nostrils by blowing the nose. *Comments:*	☐	☐	☐	
Nose Drops				
5. Follow the seven rights and three checks of safe medication administration. *Comments:*	☐	☐	☐	
6. Ask the client to lie supine and hyperextend the neck. Turn the client's head to appropriate position. *Comments:*	☐	☐	☐	
7. Squeeze some medication into the dropper. *Comments:*	☐	☐	☐	
8. Have the client exhale and occlude one nostril with a finger. *Comments:*	☐	☐	☐	
9. Insert dropper about 3/8 inch into the nostril, keeping it away from the sides of the nostril. Ask the client to inhale prescribed dosage. *Comments:*	☐	☐	☐	

continued from the previous page

Procedure 30-16	Able to Perform	Able to Perform with Assistance	Unable to Perform	Initials and Date
10. Discard any unused medication remaining in the dropper. *Comments:*	☐	☐	☐	
11. The client may blot excess drainage but may not blow the nose. Have the client remain in position for 5 minutes. *Comments:*	☐	☐	☐	
12. Repeat on other nostril if ordered. *Comments:*	☐	☐	☐	
Nasal Inhalers				
13. Repeat Actions 1–5. *Comments:*	☐	☐	☐	
14. Explain how inhalers work. *Comments:*	☐	☐	☐	
15. Have the client assume an upright position. Squeeze nose drops into dropper. *Comments:*	☐	☐	☐	
16. Have the client exhale and occlude one nostril with a finger. *Comments:*	☐	☐	☐	
17. Have the client inhale while the spray is administered. *Comments:*	☐	☐	☐	
18. Repeat the procedure on the other nostril. *Comments:*	☐	☐	☐	
19. Dispose of soiled articles appropriately. Wash hands. *Comments:*	☐	☐	☐	
20. Evaluate the effect of the medication in 15–20 minutes. *Comments:*	☐	☐	☐	
Evaluation				
1. Client is free of nasal congestion. *Comments:*	☐	☐	☐	

continued on the following page

continued from the previous page

Procedure 30-16	Able to Perform	Able to Perform with Assistance	Unable to Perform	Initials and Date
2. Client is free of nasal discharge and odor. *Comments:*	☐	☐	☐	
3. Client breathes freely through the nasal passages. *Comments:*	☐	☐	☐	
4. Client is free of sinus pain and nasal pain. *Comments:*	☐	☐	☐	
5. Client's nasal passages are moist and pink. *Comments:*	☐	☐	☐	
6. Client is free of adverse side effects secondary to the nasal medication. *Comments:*	☐	☐	☐	

Checklist for Procedure 30-17 Administering Rectal Medications

Name _____ Date _____

School _____

Instructor _____

Course _____

Procedure 30-17 Administering Rectal Medications	Able to Perform	Able to Perform with Assistance	Unable to Perform	Initials and Date
Assessment				
1. Assess the seven rights: right client, right medication, right route, right dose, right time, right to refuse, and right documentation. *Comments:*	☐	☐	☐	
2. Review the health care provider's order and identify the medication to be delivered, verifying dosage, route, time, and correct client. *Comments:*	☐	☐	☐	
3. Assess the client's need and appropriateness for rectal medication administration, and review the client's history for contraindications. *Comments:*	☐	☐	☐	
4. Consider any adjustments needed because of the client's age. *Comments:*	☐	☐	☐	
5. Observe for the desired effects or any adverse reactions, and document this response appropriately. *Comments:*	☐	☐	☐	
6. Assess the client's knowledge and understanding of the procedure. *Comments:*	☐	☐	☐	
7. Assess the client's rectal area to determine condition of skin and mucosa and presence of hemorrhoids or other rectal conditions. *Comments:*	☐	☐	☐	
Planning/Expected Outcomes				
1. The medication will be delivered appropriately and safely following the seven rights of medication administration. *Comments:*	☐	☐	☐	

continued on the following page

continued from the previous page

Procedure 30-17	Able to Perform	Able to Perform with Assistance	Unable to Perform	Initials and Date
2. The desired outcome will be verbalized by the client and documented by the nurse. *Comments:*	☐	☐	☐	
3. The treatment will be completed quickly and efficiently. *Comments:*	☐	☐	☐	
4. The client will state relief of complaint after medication administration. *Comments:*	☐	☐	☐	
Implementation				
1. Assess the client's need for the medication. *Comments:*	☐	☐	☐	
2. Check the health care provider's written order. *Comments:*	☐	☐	☐	
3. Check the medication administration record against the written order to verify the correct client, medication, route, time, and dosage. *Comments:*	☐	☐	☐	
4. Assess client for any drug allergies. *Comments:*	☐	☐	☐	
5. Review the client's history for any previous surgeries or bleeding. *Comments:*	☐	☐	☐	
6. Gather the equipment needed before entering the room. *Comments:*	☐	☐	☐	
7. Provide privacy. *Comments:*	☐	☐	☐	
8. Wash hands. *Comments:*	☐	☐	☐	
9. Ask the client to state his or her full name, and check client's identification band. *Comments:*	☐	☐	☐	

Procedure 30-17	Able to Perform	Able to Perform with Assistance	Unable to Perform	Initials and Date
10. Apply disposable gloves. *Comments:*	☐	☐	☐	
11. Assist the client into left Sim's position, with upper leg drawn up toward chest. Provide protection under the client, such as towel or pad. *Comments:*	☐	☐	☐	
12. Visually assess the client's external anus. *Comments:*	☐	☐	☐	
13. Lubricate the enema tip or remove suppository from wrapper and lubricate rounded end along with insertion finger. *Comments:*	☐	☐	☐	
14. Explain that the client will experience a cool sensation and pressure. Encourage slow, deep breaths through mouth. *Comments:*	☐	☐	☐	
15. Retract buttocks with nondominant hand, visualizing the anus. • Using the dominant index finger, slowly and gently insert the suppository through the anus, past the internal sphincter, and against the rectal wall. Depth of insertion will differ if client is a child or infant. • Gently insert the enema tip past the internal sphincter and instill the contents by slowly squeezing. *Comments:*	☐	☐	☐	
16. Remove finger or enema tip and clean the client's anal area. *Comments:*	☐	☐	☐	
17. Remove and discard gloves. *Comments:*	☐	☐	☐	
18. Wash hands. *Comments:*	☐	☐	☐	
19. Have the client remain in position for 10–15 minutes. *Comments:*	☐	☐	☐	

continued on the following page

continued from the previous page

Procedure 30-17	Able to Perform	Able to Perform with Assistance	Unable to Perform	Initials and Date
20. Place call light within reach. *Comments:*	☐	☐	☐	
21. Document administration of medication (seventh right). *Comments:*	☐	☐	☐	
22. Document effectiveness or any side effects on nursing notes. *Comments:*	☐	☐	☐	
Evaluation				
1. Medication was delivered appropriately and safely following the seven rights of medication administration. *Comments:*	☐	☐	☐	
2. The desired outcome was verbalized by the client and documented appropriately by the nurse. *Comments:*	☐	☐	☐	
3. Treatment was completed as quickly and efficiency as possible. *Comments:*	☐	☐	☐	
4. Client stated relief of complaint after medication administration. *Comments:*	☐	☐	☐	

Checklist for Procedure 30-18   Administering Vaginal Medications

Name _____ Date _____

School _____

Instructor _____

Course _____

Procedure 30-18 Administering Vaginal Medications	Able to Perform	Able to Perform with Assistance	Unable to Perform	Initials and Date
Assessment				
1. Assess the client's comfort level and symptoms. *Comments:*	☐	☐	☐	
2. Assess the client's knowledge of the purpose of the medication and treatment. *Comments:*	☐	☐	☐	
3. Assess the client's ability to self-administer the medication. *Comments:*	☐	☐	☐	
Planning/Expected Outcomes				
1. The client will experience an absence of vaginal infection, pruritus, burning, or irritation. *Comments:*	☐	☐	☐	
2. The client will experience an absence of foul-smelling, curdlike, or blood-tinged discharge. *Comments:*	☐	☐	☐	
3. The client will understand the need to perform the entire course of treatment. *Comments:*	☐	☐	☐	
4. The client will understand the importance of personal hygiene in combination with medication. *Comments:*	☐	☐	☐	
5. The client will understand the need to properly clean and store equipment. *Comments:*	☐	☐	☐	

continued on the following page

continued from the previous page

Procedure 30-18	Able to Perform	Able to Perform with Assistance	Unable to Perform	Initials and Date
Implementation				
1. Check the medication administration record against the health care provider's orders to verify the correct client, medication, route, time, and dosage. *Comments:*	☐	☐	☐	
2. Assess the client for any drug allergies. *Comments:*	☐	☐	☐	
3. Ask the client to void. *Comments:*	☐	☐	☐	
4. Check client's identification band and explain procedure before beginning. Wash hands. *Comments:*	☐	☐	☐	
5. Arrange equipment at the client's bedside. *Comments:*	☐	☐	☐	
6. Provide privacy. *Comments:*	☐	☐	☐	
7. Assist the client into a dorsal-recumbent or Sims' position. *Comments:*	☐	☐	☐	
8. Drape the client as appropriate. Provide towel or protective pad on bed. *Comments:*	☐	☐	☐	
9. Position lighting to illuminate vaginal orifice. *Comments:*	☐	☐	☐	
10. Don latex-free gloves. Assess the perineal area for redness, inflammation, discharge, or foul odor. *Comments:*	☐	☐	☐	
11. • If using an applicator, fill with medication. • If inserting a suppository, remove the suppository from the foil and position in the applicator (applicator is optional). • Apply water-soluble lubricant to suppository or applicator. *Comments:*	☐	☐	☐	

Procedure 30-18	Able to Perform	Able to Perform with Assistance	Unable to Perform	Initials and Date
12. For suppository, with nondominant hand, retract the labia. *Comments:*	☐	☐	☐	
13. With dominant hand, insert applicator 2–3 inches into the vagina, sliding the applicator posteriorly. Push the plunger to administer the medication. With a suppository, insert the tapered end first with the index finger or applicator along the posterior wall of the vagina (approximately 3 inches). *Comments:*	☐	☐	☐	
14. Withdraw the applicator and place on a towel. *Comments:*	☐	☐	☐	
15. If administering a douche or irrigation: • Warm solution to slightly above body temperature. • Position the client in a semi-recumbent position on a bedpan, on a toilet seat, or in a tub. • Apply lubricant to the irrigation nozzle and insert approximately 3 inches into the vagina. • Hang the irrigant container approximately 2 feet above the vaginal area. • Open the clamp and allow a small amount of solution to flow into the vagina. • Move the nozzle and rotate around the entire vaginal area. If the labia are inflamed, allow the solution to flow over the labia as well. If the client is on the toilet seat, alternate between closing off the labia and allowing solution to be expelled. *Comments:*	☐	☐	☐	
16. Wipe and clean the client's perineal area. *Comments:*	☐	☐	☐	
17. Apply a perineal pad. *Comments:*	☐	☐	☐	
18. Wash with warm soap and water and store the applicator in client's room. *Comments:*	☐	☐	☐	
19. Remove gloves and wash hands. *Comments:*	☐	☐	☐	

continued on the following page

continued from the previous page

Procedure 30-18	Able to Perform	Able to Perform with Assistance	Unable to Perform	Initials and Date
20. Instruct the client to remain flat for at least 30 minutes. *Comments:*	☐	☐	☐	
21. Raise side rails and place the call light within reach. *Comments:*	☐	☐	☐	
Evaluation				
1. Client experiences an absence of vaginal infection, pruritus, burning, or irritation. *Comments:*	☐	☐	☐	
2. Client experiences an absence of foul-smelling, curdlike, or blood-tinged discharge. *Comments:*	☐	☐	☐	
3. Client understands the importance of continued treatment until infection is absent. *Comments:*	☐	☐	☐	
4. Client understands the importance of personal hygiene in combination with medication. *Comments:*	☐	☐	☐	
5. Client understands the need to properly clean and store equipment. *Comments:*	☐	☐	☐	

Checklist for Procedure 30-19   Administering Nebulized Medications

Name _____ Date _____

School _____

Instructor _____

Course _____

Procedure 30-19 **Administering Nebulized Medications**	Able to Perform	Able to Perform with Assistance	Unable to Perform	Initials and Date
Assessment				
1. Assess the seven rights: right client, right medication, right route, right dose, right time, right to refuse, and right documentation. *Comments:*	☐	☐	☐	
2. Assess the client's respiratory status. *Comments:*	☐	☐	☐	
3. Evaluate the history of this episode of the client's distress. *Comments:*	☐	☐	☐	
4. Assess the client's ability to use the nebulizer or metered-dose inhaler. Determine the client's ability to understand and follow directions. *Comments:*	☐	☐	☐	
5. Assess the medication(s) currently ordered by the health care provider: action, purpose, common side effects, time of onset, and peak of action. *Comments:*	☐	☐	☐	
6. Assess the medications the client is currently taking, including over-the-counter drugs. *Comments:*	☐	☐	☐	
7. Assess the client's knowledge of the medications and use of the nebulizer or metered-dose inhaler. *Comments:*	☐	☐	☐	
8. Verify the client's drug allergy history. *Comments:*	☐	☐	☐	

continued on the following page

continued from the previous page

Procedure 30-19	Able to Perform	Able to Perform with Assistance	Unable to Perform	Initials and Date
Planning/Expected Outcomes				
1. The client will experience improved gas exchange. *Comments:*	☐	☐	☐	
2. The client's breathing pattern will become effective. *Comments:*	☐	☐	☐	
3. The client will demonstrate understanding of the need for the medication and the use of delivery system. *Comments:*	☐	☐	☐	
4. The client will not experience any adverse effects. *Comments:*	☐	☐	☐	
5. The client's anxiety level will decrease following treatment. *Comments:*	☐	☐	☐	
Implementation				
Singe-Dose Hand-Held Nebulizer 1. Assess the client's ability to use the nebulizer. *Comments:*	☐	☐	☐	
2. Check the medication administration record against the health care provider's written order to verify the correct client, medication, route, time, and dosage. *Comments:*	☐	☐	☐	
3. Assess the client for any drug allergies. *Comments:*	☐	☐	☐	
4. Check client's identification band and explain procedure before beginning. Wash hands. *Comments:*	☐	☐	☐	
5. Set up and prepare the medication(s) for one client at a time. *Comments:*	☐	☐	☐	
6. Look at the medication at eye level if using dropper to dispense the solution into the nebulizer. *Comments:*	☐	☐	☐	

Procedure 30-19	Able to Perform	Able to Perform with Assistance	Unable to Perform	Initials and Date
7. Pour the entire amount of the drug(s) into the nebulizer cup. • Avoid touching the drug while pouring into the nebulizer cup. *Comments:*	☐	☐	☐	
8. Cover the cup with the cap and fasten. *Comments:*	☐	☐	☐	
9. Fasten the T-piece to the top of the cap. *Comments:*	☐	☐	☐	
10. Fasten a short length of tubing to one end of the T-piece. *Comments:*	☐	☐	☐	
11. Fasten the mouthpiece or mask to the other end of the T-piece. *Comments:*	☐	☐	☐	
12. Identify the client prior to the administration of the medication(s). *Comments:*	☐	☐	☐	
13. Identify the medication(s) to the client and explain purpose(s) of the medication(s). *Comments:*	☐	☐	☐	
14. Advise the client to sit in an upright position. *Comments:*	☐	☐	☐	
15. Attach tubing to the bottom of the nebulizer cup. Attach the other end to the air outlet. • Adjust the air valve to 6 L/min. • Leave the air on for about 6–7 minutes until the medication is used up. *Comments:*	☐	☐	☐	
16. Instruct the client to breathe in and out slowly and deeply with lips sealed around the mouthpiece. *Comments:*	☐	☐	☐	
17. Observe that the client is using proper technique. *Comments:*	☐	☐	☐	

continued on the following page

continued from the previous page

Procedure 30-19	Able to Perform	Able to Perform with Assistance	Unable to Perform	Initials and Date
18. Wash hands. *Comments:*	☐	☐	☐	
19. When the nebulizer cup is empty: • Turn off the compressor or wall air. • Detach tubing from the air and the nebulizer cup. • If disposable, dispose of the nebulizer appropriately. • If reusable, wash, rinse, and dry the nebulizer components. *Comments:*	☐	☐	☐	
20. Immediately after the treatment, assess for results or adverse effects. *Comments:*	☐	☐	☐	
21. Reassess the client 5–10 minutes after the treatment. *Comments:*	☐	☐	☐	
22. Wash hands. *Comments:*	☐	☐	☐	
Metered-Dose Nebulizer 23. Assess the client's ability to use the metered-dose nebulizer. *Comments:*	☐	☐	☐	
24. Check the medication administration record against the health care provider's orders to verify correct client, medication, route, time, and dosage. *Comments:*	☐	☐	☐	
25. Assess the client for any drug allergies. *Comments:*	☐	☐	☐	
26. Wash hands. *Comments:*	☐	☐	☐	
27. Shake the prepackaged nebulizer. *Comments:*	☐	☐	☐	
28. Place the nebulizer into the applicator. *Comments:*	☐	☐	☐	

Procedure 30-19	Able to Perform	Able to Perform with Assistance	Unable to Perform	Initials and Date
29. Place the AeroChamber on to the nebulizer if needed. *Comments:*	☐	☐	☐	
30. Have the client exhale and place the mouthpiece in his or her mouth. *Comments:*	☐	☐	☐	
31. Have the client press down on the dispenser and simultaneously inhale slowly until lungs feel full. Hold breath for 10 seconds and exhale slowly. *Comments:*	☐	☐	☐	
32. If there is an AeroChamber attached to the nebulizer, have the client inhale slowly and deeply. *Comments:*	☐	☐	☐	
33. Observe the client to assess for possible adverse effects. *Comments:*	☐	☐	☐	
34. Have the client rinse his or her mouth. *Comments:*	☐	☐	☐	
35. Wash hands. *Comments:*	☐	☐	☐	
Evaluation				
1. Client experienced improved gas exchange. *Comments:*	☐	☐	☐	
2. Client's breathing pattern became effective. *Comments:*	☐	☐	☐	
3. Client demonstrates understanding of the need for the medication and the use of the nebulizer or metered-dose inhaler. *Comments:*	☐	☐	☐	
4. Client did not experience any adverse effects secondary to medication interactions. *Comments:*	☐	☐	☐	

continued on the following page

continued from the previous page

Procedure 30-19	Able to Perform	Able to Perform with Assistance	Unable to Perform	Initials and Date
5. Client's anxiety level decreased after treatment. *Comments:*	☐	☐	☐	

Checklist for Procedure 39-20   Applying a Dry Dressing

Name _____ Date _____

School _____

Instructor _____

Course _____

Procedure 39-20 Applying a Dry Dressing	Able to Perform	Able to Perform with Assistance	Unable to Perform	Initials and Date
Assessment				
1. Assess the client's comfort level. *Comments:*	☐	☐	☐	
2. Assess the external appearance of the initial and subsequent dressings. *Comments:*	☐	☐	☐	
3. After the dressing is removed, assess the appearance of the wound and drains. *Comments:*	☐	☐	☐	
4. Assess the client's understanding about care of the surgical site. *Comments:*	☐	☐	☐	
5. Assess the client's allergy status if solutions are to be used. *Comments:*	☐	☐	☐	
Planning/Expected Outcomes				
1. The site will be inspected for sign of infection, drainage, drainage tubes, and position of sutures or staples. *Comments:*	☐	☐	☐	
2. The initial dressing will be reinforced until changed by the health care provider. *Comments:*	☐	☐	☐	
3. The site will have the appropriate dressing applied. *Comments:*	☐	☐	☐	
4. The client/family will verbalize and/or demonstrate understanding and the ability to perform the wound care and dressing change. *Comments:*	☐	☐	☐	

continued on the following page

continued from the previous page

Procedure 39-20	**Able to Perform**	**Able to Perform with Assistance**	**Unable to Perform**	**Initials and Date**
Implementation				
1. Check client's identification band and explain procedure before beginning. Gather supplies. *Comments:*	☐	☐	☐	
2. Provide privacy. *Comments:*	☐	☐	☐	
3. Wash hands. *Comments:*	☐	☐	☐	
4. Apply clean gloves. *Comments:*	☐	☐	☐	
5. Remove dressing and place in appropriate receptacle. *Comments:*	☐	☐	☐	
6. Assess the undressed wound for signs of redness, foul odor, swelling, irritation, drainage, dehiscence, bleeding, or skin breakdown. *Comments:*	☐	☐	☐	
7. Remove used exam gloves. *Comments:*	☐	☐	☐	
8. Wash hands.. *Comments:*	☐	☐	☐	
9. Set up supplies. Open 4 × 4 gauze packages. • If incision requires cleaning, pour cleaning solution on 4 × 4 gauze pads (consult health care provider's orders and institution policy regarding cleaning incisions). *Comments:*	☐	☐	☐	
10. Apply new pair of clean gloves. *Comments:*	☐	☐	☐	

Procedure 39-20	Able to Perform	Able to Perform with Assistance	Unable to Perform	Initials and Date
11. Cleanse wound if indicated. Grasp the edges of the gauze that contains cleansing solution. • *Incision:* moving from top to bottom, clean the incision line first. Clean each side of incision using a new gauze for each wipe. • *Drain:* using a circular motion, begin at the drain site and move outward. If additional cleaning is required, obtain new gauze and clean from drain site outward. *Comments:*	☐	☐	☐	
12. Remove gloves and wash hands. *Comments:*	☐	☐	☐	
13. Apply clean gloves. *Comments:*	☐	☐	☐	
14. Apply a new dressing using 4 × 4 gauze pads folded in half to the 2 × 4 size. Place the folded gauze pad lengthwise on the wound. Tape lightly or apply tubular mesh. Initial the dressing, citing date and time it was changed. *Comments:*	☐	☐	☐	
15. Dispose of dressing appropriately, remove gloves, and then wash hands. *Comments:*	☐	☐	☐	
16. Conduct client or family education about the dressing. *Comments:*	☐	☐	☐	
Evaluation				
1. Client's comfort level was assessed during dressing change procedure. *Comments:*	☐	☐	☐	
2. Client's privacy was protected during the dressing change. *Comments:*	☐	☐	☐	
3. Correct supplies were brought in for the dressing change. *Comments:*	☐	☐	☐	
4. Client or family education was effective, as evidenced by return demonstration or verbal review. *Comments:*	☐	☐	☐	

Checklist for Procedure 39-21   Applying a Wet to Damp Dressing

Name _____ Date _____

School _____

Instructor _____

Course _____

Procedure 39-21 Applying a Wet to Damp Dressing	Able to Perform	Able to Perform with Assistance	Unable to Perform	Initials and Date
Assessment				
1. Assess the client's comfort level. *Comments:*	☐	☐	☐	
2. Assess the external appearance of the dressing. *Comments:*	☐	☐	☐	
3. After the dressing is removed, assess the appearance of the wound and drains, noting redness, swelling, purulent drainage, or ecchymosis. *Comments:*	☐	☐	☐	
4. Assess the client's understanding of the dressing changes and wound care. *Comments:*	☐	☐	☐	
5. Assess the client's healing response to previous treatments. *Comments:*	☐	☐	☐	
Planning/Expected Outcomes				
1. The site will be inspected for healing, signs of infection, and drainage. *Comments:*	☐	☐	☐	
2. The site will have the appropriate dressing applied. *Comments:*	☐	☐	☐	
3. The client or family will verbalize and/or demonstrate understanding and ability to perform the dressing change and wound care. *Comments:*	☐	☐	☐	
4. The client will experience minimal discomfort during procedure. *Comments:*	☐	☐	☐	

continued on the following page

continued from the previous page

Procedure 39-21	Able to Perform	Able to Perform with Assistance	Unable to Perform	Initials and Date
Implementation				
1. Check client's identification band and explain procedure before beginning. Review order. Gather supplies. *Comments:*	☐	☐	☐	
2. Provide privacy; draw curtains; close door. *Comments:*	☐	☐	☐	
3. Assess the need for pain medication. *Comments:*	☐	☐	☐	
4. Wash hands. *Comments:*	☐	☐	☐	
5. Apply clean gloves and other needed protective clothing. *Comments:*	☐	☐	☐	
6. Remove dressing and dispose of appropriately. Note the number of gauze pads and makeup of the old dressing. If dressing is extremely dry, a small amount of saline may be applied to that area to loosen it. *Comments:*	☐	☐	☐	
7. Observe the undressed wound for healing, signs of infection, and drainage. *Comments:*	☐	☐	☐	
8. Cleanse the skin around the incision, if necessary, with a clean, warm, wet washcloth. *Comments:*	☐	☐	☐	
9. Remove gloves and wash hands. *Comments:*	☐	☐	☐	
10. Set up supplies in a sterile field *Comments:*	☐	☐	☐	
11. Apply sterile gloves. *Comments:*	☐	☐	☐	

Procedure 39-21	Able to Perform	Able to Perform with Assistance	Unable to Perform	Initials and Date
12. Place gauze or packing material in the bowl with the ordered solution. • Wring excess solution from gauze or packing. Avoid overwringing. • Gently place wet gauze over the area. *Comments:*	☐	☐	☐	
13. Apply dry external dressing of 4 × 4 gauze pads, cover sponges, fluffs, or ABD pads. • Secure dressing with tape, Montgomery straps, or tubular mesh. *Comments:*	☐	☐	☐	
14. Remove gloves and wash hands. *Comments:*	☐	☐	☐	
15. Mark the dressing with the date, time, and initials. *Comments:*	☐	☐	☐	
16. Conduct client or family education about the dressing. *Comments:*	☐	☐	☐	
Evaluation				
1. The site was inspected for healing, signs of infection, and drainage. *Comments:*	☐	☐	☐	
2. The site had the appropriate dressing applied. *Comments:*	☐	☐	☐	
3. The client or family verbalized or demonstrated understanding and the ability, if necessary, to perform the dressing change and associated wound care. *Comments:*	☐	☐	☐	
4. The procedure was performed with minimal discomfort to the client. *Comments:*	☐	☐	☐	

Checklist for Procedure 30-22   Culturing a Wound

Name _____ Date _____

School _____

Instructor _____

Course _____

Procedure 30-22 Culturing a Wound	Able to Perform	Able to Perform with Assistance	Unable to Perform	Initials and Date
Assessment				
1. Assess the wound and the surrounding tissues for signs of infection. *Comments:*	☐	☐	☐	
2. Assess the client's overall status, including vital signs, for signs of infection such as fever, chills, or related white blood cell (WBC) count. *Comments:*	☐	☐	☐	
Planning/Expected Outcomes				
1. The culture will be collected with a minimum of pain and trauma to the client. *Comments:*	☐	☐	☐	
2. The wound culture will be representative of the wound flora, without contamination by flora outside the wound. *Comments:*	☐	☐	☐	
Implementation				
1. Check client's identification band and explain procedure before beginning. • Wash hands and apply gloves. • Remove old dressing. • Dispose of dressing and gloves appropriately. • Wash hands again. *Comments:*	☐	☐	☐	
2. Open the dressing supplies using sterile technique and apply sterile gloves. *Comments:*	☐	☐	☐	
3. Assess the wound's appearance: note quality, quantity, color, and odor of discharge. *Comments:*	☐	☐	☐	

continued on the following page

continued from the previous page

Procedure 30-22	Able to Perform	Able to Perform with Assistance	Unable to Perform	Initials and Date
4. Irrigate the wound with normal saline before collecting the culture; do not irrigate with antiseptic. *Comments:*	☐	☐	☐	
5. Blot the excess saline with a sterile gauze pad, then discard pad. *Comments:*	☐	☐	☐	
6. Remove the culture swab from the tube and gently roll the swab over the granulation tissue. Avoid eschar and wound edges. *Comments:*	☐	☐	☐	
7. • Replace the swab into the culture tube, being careful not to touch the swab to the outside of the tube. • Recap the tube. • Crush the ampule of medium located in the bottom or cap of the tube. *Comments:*	☐	☐	☐	
8. Remove gloves, wash hands, and apply sterile gloves. Dress the wound with sterile dressing. *Comments:*	☐	☐	☐	
9. Label and transport the specimen to the laboratory according to institutional policy. *Comments:*	☐	☐	☐	
10. Remove gloves and wash hands. *Comments:*	☐	☐	☐	
11. Document all assessment findings, actions taken, and that specimen was obtained. *Comments:*	☐	☐	☐	

Evaluation

	Able to Perform	Able to Perform with Assistance	Unable to Perform	Initials and Date
1. Specimen was collected with a minimum of pain or trauma to the client. *Comments:*	☐	☐	☐	
2. Wound culture is representative of the flora present in the wound, without contamination by other bacteria. *Comments:*	☐	☐	☐	

Checklist for Procedure 30-23   Irrigating a Wound

Name _____ Date _____

School _____

Instructor _____

Course _____

Procedure 30-23 Irrigating a Wound	Able to Perform	Able to Perform with Assistance	Unable to Perform	Initials and Date
Assessment				
1. Assess the current dressing. *Comments:*	☐	☐	☐	
2. Assess the client to determine if able to understand the need for the wound irrigation and cooperate with procedure. *Comments:*	☐	☐	☐	
3. Assess the client's concerns regarding this wound and the irrigation. *Comments:*	☐	☐	☐	
4. Assess the client's environment. *Comments:*	☐	☐	☐	
Planning/Expected Outcomes				
1. The wound will be free of exudate, drainage, and debris. *Comments:*	☐	☐	☐	
2. The wound will be free of signs and symptoms of infection. *Comments:*	☐	☐	☐	
3. The procedure will be performed with a minimum of trauma and pain to the client. *Comments:*	☐	☐	☐	
Implementation				
1. Check client's identification band and explain procedure before beginning. Confirm the health care provider's order for wound irrigation; note the type and strength of the ordered irrigation solution. *Comments:*	☐	☐	☐	

continued on the following page

continued from the previous page

Procedure 30-23	Able to Perform	Able to Perform with Assistance	Unable to Perform	Initials and Date
2. Assess the client's pain level and medicate if needed with analgesic 60 minutes before procedure if the medication is to be given PO or IM. *Comments:*	☐	☐	☐	
3. Assist the client onto a waterproof pad in a position that will allow the irrigant to flow from the clean to dirty areas of the wound. *Comments:*	☐	☐	☐	
4. Wash hands and apply clean gloves, gown, and mask with protective eye gear if splashes from wound fluid or blood are anticipated. Remove and discard old dressing in appropriate receptacle. *Comments:*	☐	☐	☐	
5. Assess the wound's appearance. *Comments:*	☐	☐	☐	
6. Remove gloves and wash hands. *Comments:*	☐	☐	☐	
7. Prepare the sterile irrigation tray and dressing supplies. Pour the room-temperature irrigation solution into the solution container. *Comments:*	☐	☐	☐	
8. Apply sterile gloves and new gown (and goggles if needed). *Comments:*	☐	☐	☐	
9. Position the sterile basin so that the irrigant will flow from the cleanest area to the dirtiest area and into the basin. *Comments:*	☐	☐	☐	
10. Fill the syringe or bulb syringe with irrigant and gently flush the wound. Hold the syringe approximately 1 inch above the wound bed to irrigate. Repeat until clear or the ordered amount of fluid has been used. *Comments:*	☐	☐	☐	
11. Dry the edges of the wound with sterile gauze. *Comments:*	☐	☐	☐	

Procedure 30-23	Able to Perform	Able to Perform with Assistance	Unable to Perform	Initials and Date
12. Assess the wound's appearance and drainage. *Comments:*	☐	☐	☐	
13. Apply a sterile dressing. *Comments:*	☐	☐	☐	
14. Dispose of dressings and equipment. Remove gown, mask with protective eye gear, and gloves. Wash hands. *Comments:*	☐	☐	☐	
15. Document all assessment findings and actions taken. *Comments:*	☐	☐	☐	
Evaluation				
1. Wound is free of exudates, drainage, and debris. *Comments:*	☐	☐	☐	
2. Wound is free of signs and symptoms of infection. *Comments:*	☐	☐	☐	
3. Procedure was performed with a minimum of pain or trauma to the client. *Comments:*	☐	☐	☐	

Checklist for Procedure 30-24   Administering Oxygen Therapy

Name _____ Date _____

School _____

Instructor _____

Course _____

Procedure 30-24 Administering Oxygen Therapy	Able to Perform	Able to Perform with Assistance	Unable to Perform	Initials and Date
Assessment				
1. Determine client history and acute and chronic health problems. *Comments:*	☐	☐	☐	
2. Assess the client's baseline respiratory signs, including airway, respiratory pattern, rate, depth, and rhythm, noting indications of increased work of breathing. *Comments:*	☐	☐	☐	
3. Check the extremities and mucous membranes for color. *Comments:*	☐	☐	☐	
4. Review arterial blood gas (ABG) and pulse oximetry results. *Comments:*	☐	☐	☐	
5. Note lung sounds for wheezing and crackles. *Comments:*	☐	☐	☐	
6. Assess the skin in places where tubing or equipment contacts the skin. *Comments:*	☐	☐	☐	
Planning/Expected Outcomes				
1. Oxygen levels will return to normal in blood and tissues, as evidenced by oxygen saturation ≥92% and normal skin color. *Comments:*	☐	☐	☐	
2. Respiratory rate, pattern, and depth will be within the normal range for client. *Comments:*	☐	☐	☐	
3. The client will not develop any skin or tissue irritation or breakdown. *Comments:*	☐	☐	☐	

continued on the following page

continued from the previous page

Procedure 30-24	Able to Perform	Able to Perform with Assistance	Unable to Perform	Initials and Date
4. The client will demonstrate methods to clear secretions and maintain optimal oxygenation. *Comments:*	☐	☐	☐	
5. Breathing efficiency and activity tolerance will be increased. *Comments:*	☐	☐	☐	
6. The client will understand the rationale for the therapy. *Comments:*	☐	☐	☐	

Implementation

Nasal Cannula

	Able to Perform	Able to Perform with Assistance	Unable to Perform	Initials and Date
1. Check client's identification band and explain procedure before beginning. Wash hands. *Comments:*	☐	☐	☐	
2. Verify the health care provider's order. *Comments:*	☐	☐	☐	
3. Remind clients who smoke of the reasons for not smoking while oxygen is in use. *Comments:*	☐	☐	☐	
4. If using humidity, fill humidifier to fill line with distilled water and close container. *Comments:*	☐	☐	☐	
5. Attach humidifier to oxygen flow meter. *Comments:*	☐	☐	☐	
6. Insert humidifier and flow meter into oxygen source in wall or portable unit. *Comments:*	☐	☐	☐	
7. Attach the oxygen tubing and nasal cannula to the flow meter and turn it on to the prescribed flow rate. Use extension tubing for ambulatory clients. *Comments:*	☐	☐	☐	
8. Check for bubbling in the humidifier. *Comments:*	☐	☐	☐	

Procedure 30-24	Able to Perform	Able to Perform with Assistance	Unable to Perform	Initials and Date
9. Place the nasal prongs in the client's nostrils and secure the cannula over the client's ears. Use slip ring to stabilize it under client's chin. *Comments:*	☐	☐	☐	
10. Check for proper flow rate every 4 hours and when the client returns from procedures. *Comments:*	☐	☐	☐	
11. Assess the client's nostrils every 8 hours. *Comments:*	☐	☐	☐	
12. Monitor vital signs, oxygen saturation, and client condition every 4–8 hours (or as indicated or ordered) for signs and symptoms of hypoxia. *Comments:*	☐	☐	☐	
13. Wean the client from oxygen as soon as possible using standard protocols. *Comments:*	☐	☐	☐	
Mask: Venturi (High-Flow Device), Simple Mask (Low-Flow), Partial Rebreather Mask, Nonrebreather Mask, and Face Tent				
14. Repeat Actions 1–6. *Comments:*	☐	☐	☐	
15. Attach appropriately sized mask or face tent to oxygen tubing and turn on flow meter to prescribed flow rate. Allow the reservoir bag of the nonrebreathing or partial rebreathing mask to fill completely. *Comments:*	☐	☐	☐	
16. Check for bubbling in the humidifier. *Comments:*	☐	☐	☐	
17. Place the mask or tent on the client's face and fasten snugly with elastic band. *Comments:*	☐	☐	☐	
18. Check for proper flow rate every 4 hours and when the client returns from procedures. *Comments:*	☐	☐	☐	

continued on the following page

continued from the previous page

Procedure 30-24	Able to Perform	Able to Perform with Assistance	Unable to Perform	Initials and Date
19. Ensure that the ports of the Venturi mask are not blocked. *Comments:*	☐	☐	☐	
20. Assess the client's skin for pressure areas and pad as needed. *Comments:*	☐	☐	☐	
21. Wean the client to nasal cannula and then off oxygen per protocol. *Comments:*	☐	☐	☐	
Evaluation				
1. Oxygen level returned to normal. *Comments:*	☐	☐	☐	
2. Respiratory rate, pattern, and depth are within normal range. *Comments:*	☐	☐	☐	
3. Client did not develop any skin or tissue irritation or breakdown. *Comments:*	☐	☐	☐	
4. Breathing efficiency and activity tolerance are increased. *Comments:*	☐	☐	☐	
5. Client understands the rationale for the therapy. *Comments:*	☐	☐	☐	

Checklist for Procedure 30-25   Performing Nasopharyngeal and Oropharyngeal Suctioning

Name _____ Date _____

School _____

Instructor _____

Course _____

Procedure 30-25 **Performing Nasopharyngeal and Oropharyngeal Suctioning**	Able to Perform	Able to Perform with Assistance	Unable to Perform	Initials and Date
Assessment				
1. Assess respirations for rate, rhythm, depth, and bubbling or gurgling noises. *Comments:*	☐	☐	☐	
2. Auscultate lung fields. *Comments:*	☐	☐	☐	
3. Monitor arterial blood gas and/or pulse oximetry values. *Comments:*	☐	☐	☐	
4. Assess air exchange. *Comments:*	☐	☐	☐	
5. Monitor secretions for amount, color, consistency, and odor. *Comments:*	☐	☐	☐	
6. Assess for anxiety and restlessness. *Comments:*	☐	☐	☐	
7. Assess the client's understanding of the suctioning procedure. *Comments:*	☐	☐	☐	
Planning/Expected Outcomes				
1. Client will have no coarse bubbling or gurgling noises with respirations. *Comments:*	☐	☐	☐	
2. Client will report breathing comfortably. *Comments:*	☐	☐	☐	
3. Client will have no apparent anxiety or restlessness. *Comments:*	☐	☐	☐	

continued on the following page

continued from the previous page

Procedure 30-25	Able to Perform	Able to Perform with Assistance	Unable to Perform	Initials and Date
4. Client will have arterial blood gases and pulse oximetry values within normal limits. *Comments:*	☐	☐	☐	
5. Client will express understanding of the suctioning process. *Comments:*	☐	☐	☐	
Implementation				
1. Check client's identification band and explain procedure before beginning. Choose the most appropriate route for the client. • If nasopharyngeal: inspect the nares to determine patency. *Comments:*	☐	☐	☐	
2. Advise the client that suctioning may cause coughing or gagging. *Comments:*	☐	☐	☐	
3. Wash hands. *Comments:*	☐	☐	☐	
4. Position the client in a high Fowler's or semi-Fowler's position. *Comments:*	☐	☐	☐	
5. If client is unconscious or unable to protect his or her airway, place in a side-lying position. *Comments:*	☐	☐	☐	
6. Connect extension tubing to suction device; adjust suction control to between 100 and 120 mm Hg (for adult). *Comments:*	☐	☐	☐	
7. Put on gown, mask, and goggles or face shield. *Comments:*	☐	☐	☐	
8. Using sterile technique, open the suction kit. *Comments:*	☐	☐	☐	
9. Open a packet of sterile water-soluble lubricant and squeeze out the contents onto the sterile field. *Comments:*	☐	☐	☐	

continued from the previous page

Procedure 30-25	Able to Perform	Able to Perform with Assistance	Unable to Perform	Initials and Date
10. If sterile solution is not in the kit, pour 100 mL of solution into the sterile container in the kit. *Comments:*	☐	☐	☐	
11. Lift the wrapped gloves from the kit without touching the inside of the kit or the gloves themselves. Lay the wrapped gloves next to the suction kit, open the wrapper, and put on the gloves using sterile technique. *Comments:*	☐	☐	☐	
12. If cup of sterile solution is included in the kit, open it. *Comments:*	☐	☐	☐	
13. Designate one hand as sterile and the other as clean. *Comments:*	☐	☐	☐	
14. Using your sterile hand: • Pick up the suction catheter. • Grasp the plastic connector end between your thumb and forefinger. • Coil the tip around your fingers. *Comments:*	☐	☐	☐	
15. Pick up the extension tubing with your clean hand, connect the suction catheter to the extension tubing, and do not contaminate the catheter. *Comments:*	☐	☐	☐	
16. Position your clean hand with the thumb over the catheter's suction port. *Comments:*	☐	☐	☐	
17. Dip the catheter tip into the sterile solution, activate suction, and observe the solution as it is drawn into the catheter. *Comments:*	☐	☐	☐	
18. For oropharyngeal suctioning: • Ask the client to open his or her mouth. • Without activating the suction, use the sterile hand to insert the catheter. • Advance catheter until a pool of secretions is reached or the client coughs. • Do not poke catheter in oropharynx. *Comments:*	☐	☐	☐	

continued on the following page

continued from the previous page

Procedure 30-25	Able to Perform	Able to Perform with Assistance	Unable to Perform	Initials and Date
19. For nasopharyngeal suctioning: • Estimate the distance from the tip of the client's nose to the earlobe. • Grasp the catheter between your thumb and forefinger at a point equal to this distance from the catheter tip. *Comments:*	☐	☐	☐	
20. Dip the tip of the catheter into the water-soluble lubricant and coat catheter tip liberally. *Comments:*	☐	☐	☐	
21. Use sterile hand to insert the catheter into the nostril with the suction control port uncovered. Advance the catheter with a slight downward slant to the point marked by your thumb and forefinger. Slight rotation of the catheter may be used to ease insertion. *Comments:*	☐	☐	☐	
22. If resistance is met, do not force the catheter. Withdraw the catheter and attempt insertion via opposite nostril. *Comments:*	☐	☐	☐	
23. With clean hand, apply suction by occluding the suction control port with your thumb; at the same time, slowly rotate the catheter by rolling it between your thumb and fingers while withdrawing it. Apply suction for no longer than 15 seconds at a time. *Comments:*	☐	☐	☐	
24. Repeat Action 23 until secretions have been cleared; allow brief rest periods between suctioning episodes. *Comments:*	☐	☐	☐	
25. Withdraw catheter by looping it around your fingers as you pull it out. *Comments:*	☐	☐	☐	
26. Dip the catheter into the sterile solution and apply suction. *Comments:*	☐	☐	☐	
27. Disconnect the catheter from the extension tubing. Holding the coiled catheter in the gloved hand, remove glove by pulling it over the catheter. Discard catheter and glove in an appropriate container. *Comments:*	☐	☐	☐	

Procedure 30-25	Able to Perform	Able to Perform with Assistance	Unable to Perform	Initials and Date
28. Discard remaining supplies in the appropriate container and wash hands. *Comments:*	☐	☐	☐	
29. Provide the client with oral hygiene if needed or desired. *Comments:*	☐	☐	☐	
Evaluation				
1. Client has no bubbling or gurgling sounds with breathing. *Comments:*	☐	☐	☐	
2. Client has no signs of or reports no dyspnea or distress. *Comments:*	☐	☐	☐	
3. Client has no apparent anxiety or restlessness. *Comments:*	☐	☐	☐	
4. Arterial blood gases and/or pulse oximetry values are within normal limits. *Comments:*	☐	☐	☐	
5. Client is able to verbalize understanding of suctioning process. *Comments:*	☐	☐	☐	

Checklist for Procedure 30-26   Performing Tracheostomy Care

Name _____ Date _____

School _____

Instructor _____

Course _____

Procedure 30-26 Performing Tracheostomy Care	Able to Perform	Able to Perform with Assistance	Unable to Perform	Initials and Date
Assessment				
1. Assess respirations for rate, rhythm, and depth. *Comments:*	☐	☐	☐	
2. Assess the client's lung sounds. *Comments:*	☐	☐	☐	
3. Assess the client's arterial blood gases and pulse oximetry values. *Comments:*	☐	☐	☐	
4. Assess the movement of air through the tracheostomy tube. *Comments:*	☐	☐	☐	
5. Assess the amount and color of tracheal secretions. *Comments:*	☐	☐	☐	
6. Assess for anxiety, restlessness, and fear. *Comments:*	☐	☐	☐	
7. Assess the client's understanding of the procedure. *Comments:*	☐	☐	☐	
8. Assess the area around the tracheostomy for redness, swelling, and drainage. *Comments:*	☐	☐	☐	
Planning/Expected Outcomes				
1. The client's airway will be free of obstruction. *Comments:*	☐	☐	☐	
2. The procedure will be performed with a minimum of client anxiety. *Comments:*	☐	☐	☐	

continued on the following page

continued from the previous page

Procedure 30-26	Able to Perform	Able to Perform with Assistance	Unable to Perform	Initials and Date
3. The client's skin will remain intact and free of redness and excoriation. *Comments:*	☐	☐	☐	
4. The client will remain free of symptoms of infection. *Comments:*	☐	☐	☐	
5. The client will have cannulas free of secretions and clean, secure ties. *Comments:*	☐	☐	☐	
Implementation				
1. Check client's identification band and explain procedure before beginning. Wash hands and apply clean gloves. *Comments:*	☐	☐	☐	
2. Remove soiled dressing and discard. *Comments:*	☐	☐	☐	
Conventional/Reusable Inner Cannula				
3. Open tracheostomy care set. *Comments:*	☐	☐	☐	
4. Place hydrogen peroxide solution and sterile water or saline in separate basins. *Comments:*	☐	☐	☐	
5. Apply sterile gloves. *Comments:*	☐	☐	☐	
6. Dip applicator in the basin of hydrogen peroxide. *Comments:*	☐	☐	☐	
7. Remove inner cannula. *Comments:*	☐	☐	☐	
8. Place inner cannula in basin of hydrogen peroxide. *Comments:*	☐	☐	☐	

Procedure 30-26	Able to Perform	Able to Perform with Assistance	Unable to Perform	Initials and Date
9. Clean the area under the neck plate of the tracheostomy tube using a cotton applicator moistened with hydrogen peroxide. *Comments:*	☐	☐	☐	
10. Rinse area under the neck plate with a cotton applicator moistened with sterile water or saline. *Comments:*	☐	☐	☐	
11. Dry skin under the neck plate with a cotton-tipped applicator. *Comments:*	☐	☐	☐	
12. Apply tracheostomy gauze under neck plate of tube. (Change frequently to prevent infection and skin breakdown.) *Comments:*	☐	☐	☐	
13. Use a tracheostomy brush or sterile cotton-tipped applicator to clean inner cannula. *Comments:*	☐	☐	☐	
14. Rinse inner cannula with sterile water or sterile saline. *Comments:*	☐	☐	☐	
15. Dry inner cannula. *Comments:*	☐	☐	☐	
16. Reinsert inner cannula and lock it into place. *Comments:*	☐	☐	☐	
17. Remove gloves and wash hands. *Comments:*	☐	☐	☐	
Disposable Inner Cannula				
18. Wash hands. Open disposable cannula without touching cannula. *Comments:*	☐	☐	☐	
19. Apply sterile gloves. *Comments:*	☐	☐	☐	

continued on the following page

continued from the previous page

Procedure 30-26	Able to Perform	Able to Perform with Assistance	Unable to Perform	Initials and Date
20. Remove used inner cannula and discard. *Comments:*	☐	☐	☐	
21. Replace inner cannula with new disposable cannula. *Comments:*	☐	☐	☐	
22. Remove gloves and wash hands. *Comments:*	☐	☐	☐	
Two-Person Technique of Changing Tracheostomy Ties				
23. Cut two pieces of twill tape about 12–14 inches in length. *Comments:*	☐	☐	☐	
24. Fold about 1 inch below the end of twill tape and cut a half-inch slit lengthwise in the center of the fold. Repeat for other tape. *Comments:*	☐	☐	☐	
25. Have second person hold the tracheostomy tube in place with fingers on both sides of the neck plate. *Comments:*	☐	☐	☐	
26. Untie old tracheostomy ties and discard. *Comments:*	☐	☐	☐	
27. Insert the split end of the twill tape through the opening on one side of the neck plate. Pull the distal end of the tie through the cut and pull tightly. *Comments:*	☐	☐	☐	
28. Repeat procedure with second piece of twill tape. *Comments:*	☐	☐	☐	
29. Tie tracheostomy tapes with a double knot at the side of the neck. *Comments:*	☐	☐	☐	
30. Insert one finger under tracheostomy tapes. *Comments:*	☐	☐	☐	
31. Insert tracheostomy gauze under neck plate of tube. *Comments:*	☐	☐	☐	

Procedure 30-26	Able to Perform	Able to Perform with Assistance	Unable to Perform	Initials and Date
32. Discard all used materials and wash hands. *Comments:*	☐	☐	☐	
33. Follow Actions 22–23 and 26–28. *Comments:*	☐	☐	☐	
34. Hold the neck plate firmly with one hand; untie and remove old tracheostomy tapes and discard. *Comments:*	☐	☐	☐	
35. Place one finger under tracheostomy ties. *Comments:*	☐	☐	☐	
36. Discard all used materials and wash hands. *Comments:*	☐	☐	☐	
Evaluation				
1. Client's airway is free of obstruction. *Comments:*	☐	☐	☐	
2. Client anxiety was minimal during procedure. *Comments:*	☐	☐	☐	
3. There is no evidence of infection. *Comments:*	☐	☐	☐	
4. Airway remains patent. *Comments:*	☐	☐	☐	
5. Cannulas are free of secretions and have clean, secured ties. *Comments:*	☐	☐	☐	
6. Client's skin remained intact and free of redness and excoriation. *Comments:*	☐	☐	☐	

Checklist for Procedure 30-27   Performing Tracheostomy Suctioning

Name _____ Date _____

School _____

Instructor _____

Course _____

Procedure 30-27 **Performing Tracheostomy Suctioning**	**Able to Perform**	**Able to Perform with Assistance**	**Unable to Perform**	**Initials and Date**
Assessment				
1. Assess respirations for rate, rhythm, and depth. *Comments:*	☐	☐	☐	
2. Auscultate lung fields. *Comments:*	☐	☐	☐	
3. Monitor arterial blood gases and/or pulse oximetry values. *Comments:*	☐	☐	☐	
4. Assess passage of air through the tracheostomy tube. *Comments:*	☐	☐	☐	
5. Monitor secretions for amount, color, consistency, and odor. *Comments:*	☐	☐	☐	
6. Assess for anxiety and restlessness. *Comments:*	☐	☐	☐	
7. Assess the client's understanding of the suctioning procedure. *Comments:*	☐	☐	☐	
Planning/Expected Outcomes				
1. The client will have no crackles or wheezes in large airways and no cyanosis. *Comments:*	☐	☐	☐	
2. The client will report breathing comfortably and will have no apparent anxiety or restlessness. *Comments:*	☐	☐	☐	
3. The client will have minimal amount of thin, normal-colored secretions. *Comments:*	☐	☐	☐	

continued on the following page

continued from the previous page

Procedure 30-27	Able to Perform	Able to Perform with Assistance	Unable to Perform	Initials and Date
4. The client will maintain a patent airway. *Comments:*	☐	☐	☐	
5. The client will maintain adequate pulse oximetry. *Comments:*	☐	☐	☐	
Implementation				
1. Check client's identification band and explain procedure before beginning. Assess depth and rate of respirations and breath sounds. *Comments:*	☐	☐	☐	
2. Assemble supplies on bedside table. *Comments:*	☐	☐	☐	
3. Wash hands. *Comments:*	☐	☐	☐	
4. Position the client in high Fowler's or semi-Fowler's position. *Comments:*	☐	☐	☐	
5. Connect extension tubing to suction device and adjust suction control to between 100 and 120 mm Hg. *Comments:*	☐	☐	☐	
6. Put on gown, mask, and goggles or face shield. *Comments:*	☐	☐	☐	
7. Using sterile technique, open the tracheostomy care kit. Consider spreading the inner wrapper of kit as a sterile field. Add sterile suction if not in kit. *Comments:*	☐	☐	☐	
8. Lift wrapped gloves from the kit without touching the inside of the kit or the gloves themselves. Lay the gloves down, open the wrapper and put on the gloves using sterile gloving technique. *Comments:*	☐	☐	☐	
9. Pour hydrogen peroxide in one basin and sterile water or saline in the other. *Comments:*	☐	☐	☐	

continued from the previous page

Procedure 30-27	Able to Perform	Able to Perform with Assistance	Unable to Perform	Initials and Date
10. Designate one hand as sterile and the other as clean. *Comments:*	☐	☐	☐	
11. Using your sterile hand, pick up the suction catheter. Grasp the plastic connector end between your thumb and forefinger and coil the tip around your remaining fingers. *Comments:*	☐	☐	☐	
12. Pick up the extension tubing with your clean hand. Connect the suction catheter to the extension tubing. Do not contaminate the catheter. *Comments:*	☐	☐	☐	
13. Administer oxygen or use Ambu bag with clean hand before beginning. *Comments:*	☐	☐	☐	
14. Remove inner cannula and place in basin of hydrogen peroxide to loosen secretions, if reusable, or set aside if disposable. Do not dispose of disposable cannula until new inner cannula is securely in place. *Comments:*	☐	☐	☐	
15. Position your clean hand with the thumb over the catheter's suction port, dip the catheter tip into the sterile solution, and activate the suction. Observe the solution drawn into the catheter. *Comments:*	☐	☐	☐	
16. Remove thumb from suction port. *Comments:*	☐	☐	☐	
17. Using your clean hand, remove the oxygen delivery device from the tracheostomy tube and place it on a clean surface. *Comments:*	☐	☐	☐	
18. Without occluding the suction control port, insert the catheter tip into the tracheostomy tube and advance it until the client coughs or resistance is met, then withdraw slightly. *Comments:*	☐	☐	☐	

continued on the following page

continued from the previous page

Procedure 30-27	Able to Perform	Able to Perform with Assistance	Unable to Perform	Initials and Date
19. Apply suction by occluding the suction control port with your thumb while rotating the catheter and slowly withdrawing it. Apply suction no longer than 15 seconds at a time. *Comments:*	☐	☐	☐	
20. Repeat Action 19 until all secretions have been cleared; allow brief rest periods between suctioning episodes. Encourage client to breathe deeply between suctioning episodes. Provide oxygen between phases of the suction catheter. *Comments:*	☐	☐	☐	
21. Withdraw catheter and dip it into the cup of sterile saline, applying suction. *Comments:*	☐	☐	☐	
22. Clean inner cannula using tracheostomy brush and rinse well in sterile water or sterile saline. Dry (or open new disposable inner cannula). *Comments:*	☐	☐	☐	
23. Reinsert inner cannula and lock into place. *Comments:*	☐	☐	☐	
24. Reapply oxygen delivery device. *Comments:*	☐	☐	☐	
25. Dip the catheter tip into the sterile solution and apply suction. *Comments:*	☐	☐	☐	
26. Disconnect the catheter from the extension tubing. Discard catheter and gloves in the appropriate container. *Comments:*	☐	☐	☐	
27. Discard remaining supplies in the appropriate container. *Comments:*	☐	☐	☐	
28. Wash hands. *Comments:*	☐	☐	☐	
29. Provide the client with oral hygiene if indicated or desired. *Comments:*	☐	☐	☐	

Procedure 30-27	Able to Perform	Able to Perform with Assistance	Unable to Perform	Initials and Date
Evaluation				
1. Airway is patent and free of obstruction. *Comments:*	☐	☐	☐	
2. Client anxiety was minimal during procedure. *Comments:*	☐	☐	☐	
3. Arterial blood gases and pulse oximetry values have improved. *Comments:*	☐	☐	☐	
4. There is no evidence of infection. *Comments:*	☐	☐	☐	
5. Client's breathing is easier. Client shows no signs of dyspnea or distress. *Comments:*	☐	☐	☐	
6. Cannulas are free of secretions and have clean, secured ties. *Comments:*	☐	☐	☐	
7. Client's skin remained intact and free of redness and excoriation. *Comments:*	☐	☐	☐	

Checklist for Procedure 30-28   Postoperative Exercise Instruction

Name _____ Date _____

School _____

Instructor _____

Course _____

Procedure 30-28 Postoperative Exercise Instruction	Able to Perform	Able to Perform with Assistance	Unable to Perform	Initials and Date
Assessment				
1. Assess the client's current understanding of postoperative procedures. *Comments:*	☐	☐	☐	
2. Assess the client's ability to understand the postoperative exercise instructions. *Comments:*	☐	☐	☐	
3. Assess client limitations that would prevent or impair the performance of postoperative exercises. *Comments:*	☐	☐	☐	
Planning/Expected Outcomes				
1. The client will be able to successfully demonstrate postoperative exercises, deep breathing, coughing, pillow splinting, turning and proper body alignment, leg and foot exercises, and out-of-bed transfers. *Comments:*	☐	☐	☐	
2. The client will be able to successfully demonstrate proper use of the incentive spirometer. *Comments:*	☐	☐	☐	
Implementation				
1. Check the client's identification band, wash hands, and organize equipment. *Comments:*	☐	☐	☐	
2. Apply gloves. *Comments:*	☐	☐	☐	
3. Place the client in a sitting position. *Comments:*	☐	☐	☐	

continued on the following page

continued from the previous page

Procedure 30-28	Able to Perform	Able to Perform with Assistance	Unable to Perform	Initials and Date
4. Demonstrate deep breathing exercises. • Place one hand on abdomen during inhalation. • Expand the abdomen and rib cage on inspiration. • Inhale slowly and evenly through your nose until you achieve maximum chest expansion. • Hold breath for 2–3 seconds. • Slowly exhale through your mouth until maximum chest contraction has been achieved. *Comments:*	☐	☐	☐	
5. Have the client return-demonstrate the deep breathing exercises and repeat 3–4 times. *Comments:*	☐	☐	☐	
6. Instruct the client on the use of an incentive spirometer. • Hold the volume-oriented spirometer upright. • Exhale; seal lips tightly around the mouthpiece; take a slow deep breath to elevate the balls in the plastic tube. Hold the inspiration for at least 3 seconds. • The client measures the amount of inspired air volume on the calibrated plastic tube. • Remove the mouthpiece and exhale normally. • Take several normal breaths. *Comments:*	☐	☐	☐	
7. Have the client repeat the procedure 4–5 times. *Comments:*	☐	☐	☐	
8. Have the client cough after the incentive effort. *Comments:*	☐	☐	☐	
9. Demonstrate splinting and coughing. • Have the client slowly raise head and sniff the air. • Have the client bend forward and exhale slowly through pursed lips. • Repeat breathing 2–3 times. • When the client is ready to cough, place a folded pillow against the abdomen and hold with clasped hands. • Have the client take a deep breath and begin coughing immediately after inspiration is completed by bending forward slightly and producing a series of soft, staccato coughs. • Have a tissue ready. *Comments:*	☐	☐	☐	
10. Have the client return-demonstrate splinting and coughing. *Comments:*	☐	☐	☐	

Procedure 30-28	Able to Perform	Able to Perform with Assistance	Unable to Perform	Initials and Date
11. Wash the incentive spirometer mouthpiece and store in a clean container. Change disposable mouthpieces every 24 hours. *Comments:*	☐	☐	☐	
12. Teach the client leg and foot exercises. • With heels on bed, push toes of both feet toward the foot of the bed until the calf muscles tighten, then relax feet. Pull the toes toward the chin until calf muscles tighten; then relax feet. • With heels on bed, lift and circle both ankles, first to the right and then to the left; repeat 3 times, relax. • Flex and extend each knee alternately, sliding foot up along the bed; relax. *Comments:*	☐	☐	☐	
13. Have the client return-demonstrate the leg and foot exercises. *Comments:*	☐	☐	☐	
14. Explain how to turn in bed and get out of bed. *Comments:*	☐	☐	☐	
15. Clients with a left-sided abdominal or chest incision should turn to the right side of bed and sit up as follows: • Flex the knees. • With the right hand, splint the incision with hand or small pillow. • Turn toward right side by pushing with the left foot and grasping the nurse or side rail of the bed with the left hand. • Sit up on the side of the bed using the left arm and hand to push down against the mattress or side rail. *Comments:*	☐	☐	☐	
16. Reverse instructions in Action 15 for clients with a right-sided incision. *Comments:*	☐	☐	☐	
17. Instruct clients who have had orthopedic surgery how to use an overhead trapeze. *Comments:*	☐	☐	☐	
18. Wash hands. *Comments:*	☐	☐	☐	

continued on the following page

continued from the previous page

Procedure 30-28	Able to Perform	Able to Perform with Assistance	Unable to Perform	Initials and Date
Evaluation				
1. Client successfully demonstrated postoperative exercises, deep breathing, coughing, pillow splinting, turning and proper body alignment, leg and foot exercises, and out-of-bed transfers. *Comments:*	☐	☐	☐	
2. Client successfully demonstrated proper use of incentive spirometer. *Comments:*	☐	☐	☐	

Checklist for Procedure 30-29   Performing a Skin Puncture

Name _____ Date _____

School _____

Instructor _____

Course _____

Procedure 30-29 Performing a Skin Puncture	Able to Perform	Able to Perform with Assistance	Unable to Perform	Initials and Date
Assessment				
1. Assess the condition of the client's skin at the potential puncture site. *Comments:*	☐	☐	☐	
2. Assess the circulation at the potential puncture site. *Comments:*	☐	☐	☐	
3. Assess the client's comfort level regarding the procedure. *Comments:*	☐	☐	☐	
4. Assess the cleanliness of the client's skin. *Comments:*	☐	☐	☐	
Planning/Expected Outcomes				
1. An adequate blood specimen will be obtained. *Comments:*	☐	☐	☐	
2. The client will suffer minimal trauma during specimen collection. *Comments:*	☐	☐	☐	
3. The specimen will be collected and stored in a manner compatible with the ordered tests. *Comments:*	☐	☐	☐	
Implementation				
1. Wash hands. *Comments:*	☐	☐	☐	
2. Check client's identification band, if appropriate. *Comments:*	☐	☐	☐	

continued on the following page

continued from the previous page

Procedure 30-29	Able to Perform	Able to Perform with Assistance	Unable to Perform	Initials and Date
3. Explain procedure to client. *Comments:*	☐	☐	☐	
4. Prepare supplies, open packages, label specimen tubes, and place in easy reach. *Comments:*	☐	☐	☐	
5. Apply gloves. *Comments:*	☐	☐	☐	
6. Select site: lateral aspect of the fingertips in adults and children; heel for neonates and infants. *Comments:*	☐	☐	☐	
7. Place the hand or heel in a dependent position; apply warm compresses if fingers or heel are cool to touch. *Comments:*	☐	☐	☐	
8. Place hand towel or absorbent pad under the extremity. *Comments:*	☐	☐	☐	
9. Cleanse puncture site with an antiseptic and allow to dry. *Comments:*	☐	☐	☐	
10. With nondominant hand, apply light, milking pressure above or around the puncture site. Do not touch the puncture site. *Comments:*	☐	☐	☐	
11. With the sterile lancet at a 90-degree angle to the skin, use a quick stab to puncture the skin. • Automatic unistik: push lancet into body of unistik until it clicks. Hold body of the unistik and twist off the lancet cap. Place the end of unistik tightly against the client's finger and press the lever. *Comments:*	☐	☐	☐	
12. Wipe off the first drop of blood with sterile gauze; allow the blood to flow freely. *Comments:*	☐	☐	☐	
13. Collect the blood into the appropriate tube(s). *Comments:*	☐	☐	☐	

Procedure 30-29	Able to Perform	Able to Perform with Assistance	Unable to Perform	Initials and Date
14. Apply pressure to the puncture site with sterile gauze. *Comments:*	☐	☐	☐	
15. Place contaminated articles into a sharps container. *Comments:*	☐	☐	☐	
16. Remove and dispose of gloves. Wash hands. *Comments:*	☐	☐	☐	
17. Position the client for comfort with call light within reach. *Comments:*	☐	☐	☐	
18. Wash hands. *Comments:*	☐	☐	☐	
Evaluation				
1. Specimen was adequate. *Comments:*	☐	☐	☐	
2. Client did not sustain any trauma. *Comments:*	☐	☐	☐	

Checklist for Procedure 30-30   Feeding and Medicating via Enteral Tube

Name _____ Date _____

School _____

Instructor _____

Course _____

Procedure 30-30 **Feeding and Medicating via Enteral Tube**	Able to Perform	Able to Perform with Assistance	Unable to Perform	Initials and Date
Assessment				
1. Assess the client for signs of gastric distress, such as nausea, vomiting, and cramping. *Comments:*	☐	☐	☐	
2. Assess the feeding tube placement every 4 hours. *Comments:*	☐	☐	☐	
3. Assess the client's respiratory status. *Comments:*	☐	☐	☐	
4. Assess the client's ongoing nutritional status. *Comments:*	☐	☐	☐	
5. Assess the client's intake and output. *Comments:*	☐	☐	☐	
Planning/Expected Outcomes				
1. The client will receive the correct volume and formula over the correct time period. *Comments:*	☐	☐	☐	
2. The client will not experience any undesirable effects: aspiration, nausea, vomiting, abdominal distention, cramping, diarrhea, or constipation. *Comments:*	☐	☐	☐	
3. The client's weight and nutritional status will remain stable or improve. *Comments:*	☐	☐	☐	
4. The client will not experience any adverse skin or gastrointestinal effects. *Comments:*	☐	☐	☐	

continued on the following page

continued from the previous page

Procedure 30-30	Able to Perform	Able to Perform with Assistance	Unable to Perform	Initials and Date
Implementation				
1. Review the client's medical record for formula, amount, and time. *Comments:*	☐	☐	☐	
2. Wash hands. Gather equipment and formula. *Comments:*	☐	☐	☐	
3. Identify client by checking arm band. *Comments:*	☐	☐	☐	
4. Explain procedure to client. *Comments:*	☐	☐	☐	
5. Assemble equipment. Add color to formula if used. Fill bag with prescribed amount of formula. *Comments:*	☐	☐	☐	
6. Place the client on right side in a high-Fowler's position. *Comments:*	☐	☐	☐	
7. Provide for privacy. *Comments:*	☐	☐	☐	
8. Wash hands and don nonsterile gloves. *Comments:*	☐	☐	☐	
9. Observe for abdominal distension; auscultate for bowel sounds. *Comments:*	☐	☐	☐	
10. Aspirate stomach for residual contents by inserting syringe into adapter port and aspirating. If residual contents are greater than 50–100 mL (or in accordance with agency policy), hold feeding. Instill aspirated contents back into stomach. *Comments:*	☐	☐	☐	
11. Administer tube feeding. *Comments:*	☐	☐	☐	

Procedure 30-30	Able to Perform	Able to Perform with Assistance	Unable to Perform	Initials and Date
Intermittent Bolus				
12. Pinch the tubing. *Comments:*	☐	☐	☐	
13. Remove plunger from barrel of syringe and attach to adapter. *Comments:*	☐	☐	☐	
14. Fill syringe with formula. *Comments:*	☐	☐	☐	
15. Infuse slowly; add formula to syringe until prescribed amount has been administered. *Comments:*	☐	☐	☐	
16. Flush tubing with 30–60 mL or prescribed amount of water. *Comments:*	☐	☐	☐	
17. Remove syringe and replace cap into adapter port. *Comments:*	☐	☐	☐	
Intermittent Gavage Feeding				
18. Hang bag on IV pole 18 inches above the client's head. *Comments:*	☐	☐	☐	
19. Fill bag with ordered amount of feeding. Remove air from tubing by opening clamp on tubing and allow feeding to flow through tubing. *Comments:*	☐	☐	☐	
20. Attach distal end of tubing to feeding tube adapter and adjust drip rate to infuse over prescribed time. *Comments:*	☐	☐	☐	
21. When bag empties of formula, infuse 30–60 mL or prescribed amount of water; close clamp. *Comments:*	☐	☐	☐	
22. Remove tubing from adapter port and cap adapter port. *Comments:*	☐	☐	☐	

continued on the following page

continued from the previous page

Procedure 30-30	Able to Perform	Able to Perform with Assistance	Unable to Perform	Initials and Date
23. Change bags every 24 hours. *Comments:*	☐	☐	☐	
Continuous Gavage				
24. Check tube placement at least every 4 hours. *Comments:*	☐	☐	☐	
25. Check residual at least every 4 hours. *Comments:*	☐	☐	☐	
26. If residual is greater than 100 mL, stop feeding. *Comments:*	☐	☐	☐	
27. Add formula to bag for a 4-hour period; dilute with water if prescribed. *Comments:*	☐	☐	☐	
28. Hang gavage bag on IV pole. Prime tubing. *Comments:*	☐	☐	☐	
29. Thread tubing through feeding pump and attach distal end of tubing to feeding tube adapter. *Comments:*	☐	☐	☐	
30. Program rate. *Comments:*	☐	☐	☐	
31. Monitor infusion rate and signs of respiratory distress or diarrhea. *Comments:*	☐	☐	☐	
32. Flush tube with water every 4 hours or as prescribed, or following administration of medications. *Comments:*	☐	☐	☐	
33. Replace disposable feeding bag at least every 24 hours. *Comments:*	☐	☐	☐	
34. Elevate head of bed at least 30 degrees at all times and turn client every 2 hours. *Comments:*	☐	☐	☐	

continued from the previous page

Procedure 30-30	Able to Perform	Able to Perform with Assistance	Unable to Perform	Initials and Date
35. Provide oral hygiene every 2–4 hours. *Comments:*	☐	☐	☐	
36. Administer water as prescribed, with and between feedings. *Comments:*	☐	☐	☐	
37. Remove gloves and wash hands. *Comments:*	☐	☐	☐	
Instilling Medications into Enteral Tubes				
38. Wash hands and don gloves. *Comments:*	☐	☐	☐	
39. Assist the client to high- or semi-Fowler's position. *Comments:*	☐	☐	☐	
40. Place linen saver over bed linen. *Comments:*	☐	☐	☐	
41. Verify nasogastic tube placement. *Comments:*	☐	☐	☐	
42. Attach syringe to tube and pour 30 mL of prepared medication into syringe. *Comments:*	☐	☐	☐	
43. Open clamp on tube. *Comments:*	☐	☐	☐	
44. Hold syringe at a slight angle; add more medication before syringe empties. *Comments:*	☐	☐	☐	
45. For two or more medications, give each separately, with 5-mL water rinse between medications. *Comments:*	☐	☐	☐	
46. As syringe empties with the last of the medication, slowly add 30–50 mL water. *Comments:*	☐	☐	☐	

continued on the following page

continued from the previous page

Procedure 30-30	Able to Perform	Able to Perform with Assistance	Unable to Perform	Initials and Date
47. Before tube empties of water, clamp tube, detach and dispose of the syringe. *Comments:*	☐	☐	☐	
48. Place clients with a nasogastic tube on the right side, with head slightly elevated, for 30 minutes. *Comments:*	☐	☐	☐	
49. Remove gloves and wash hands. *Comments:*	☐	☐	☐	
Evaluation				
1. Client received the correct feeding formula and the correct volume of formula over the correct time period. *Comments:*	☐	☐	☐	
2. Client did not experience any undesirable effects, such as aspiration, nausea, vomiting, abdominal distention, cramping, diarrhea, or constipation. *Comments:*	☐	☐	☐	
3. Client's weight and nutritional status remained stable or improved. *Comments:*	☐	☐	☐	
4. Client did not experience any adverse skin or gastrointestinal effects from the tube. *Comments:*	☐	☐	☐	

Checklist for Procedure 31-1   Inserting and Maintaining a Nasogastric Tube

Name _____ Date _____

School _____

Instructor _____

Course _____

Procedure 31-1 **Inserting and Maintaining a Nasogastric Tube**	Able to Perform	Able to Perform with Assistance	Unable to Perform	Initials and Date
Assessment				
1. Assess the client's consciousness level. *Comments:*	☐	☐	☐	
2. Check the client's chart for any history of nostril surgery, injury, or unusual nostril bleeding. *Comments:*	☐	☐	☐	
3. Use a penlight to assess nostrils for a deviated septum. *Comments:*	☐	☐	☐	
4. Ask the client to breathe, occluding one nostril at a time. *Comments:*	☐	☐	☐	
5. Assess for latex allergy. *Comments:*	☐	☐	☐	
Planning/Expected Outcomes				
1. The client's nutritional status will improve. *Comments:*	☐	☐	☐	
2. The client's nutritional needs will be met with assistance of tube feeding. *Comments:*	☐	☐	☐	
3. The client will maintain a patent airway. *Comments:*	☐	☐	☐	
4. The client will not have diarrhea caused by nasogastric (NG) feeding. *Comments:*	☐	☐	☐	
5. Mouth mucous membranes will remain moist and intact. *Comments:*	☐	☐	☐	

continued on the following page

continued from the previous page

Procedure 31-1	Able to Perform	Able to Perform with Assistance	Unable to Perform	Initials and Date
6. The client will maintain a normal fluid volume. *Comments:*	☐	☐	☐	
7. The client's comfort level will increase. *Comments:*	☐	☐	☐	
8. Skin around the tube will remain intact with no redness or blisters. *Comments:*	☐	☐	☐	
Implementation				
1. Review client's medical history for conditions that have resulted in a loss of the gag reflex. *Comments:*	☐	☐	☐	
2. Check client's identification arm band. Assess client's consciousness and ability to understand. Explain the procedure and develop a hand signal. *Comments:*	☐	☐	☐	
3. Provide privacy. Prepare the equipment. *Comments:*	☐	☐	☐	
4. Prepare the environment; place the bed in a high-Fowler's position. Cover the client's chest with a towel. *Comments:*	☐	☐	☐	
5. Wash hands and don gloves and personal protective equipment. *Comments:*	☐	☐	☐	
6. Assess the client's nostrils with a pen light and have client blow nose one nostril at a time. *Comments:*	☐	☐	☐	
7. Measure the distance from the tip of the nose to the earlobe and then to the xiphoid process of the sternum. Mark this distance with a piece of tape. *Comments:*	☐	☐	☐	

Procedure 31-1	Able to Perform	Able to Perform with Assistance	Unable to Perform	Initials and Date
8. Lubricate first 4 inches of the tube with water-soluble lubricant. *Comments:*	☐	☐	☐	
9. Ask the client to slightly flex the neck backward. *Comments:*	☐	☐	☐	
10. Gently insert the tube into a naris. *Comments:*	☐	☐	☐	
11. Tip the client's head forward once the tube reaches the nasopharynx. If the client continues to gag, stop a moment. *Comments:*	☐	☐	☐	
12. Advance the tube several inches at a time as the client swallows. If gag reflex is present, have the client swallow water or ice chips as tube is advanced *Comments:*	☐	☐	☐	
13. Withdraw the tube immediately if there are signs of respiratory distress. *Comments:*	☐	☐	☐	
14. Advance the tube until the taped mark is reached. *Comments:*	☐	☐	☐	
15. Split a 4-inch strip of tape lengthwise 2 inches. Secure the tube with the tape by placing the wide portion of the tape on the bridge of the nose and wrapping the split ends around the tube. Tape to cheek as well if desired. *Comments:*	☐	☐	☐	
16. Check the placement of the tube: • Aspirate gastric content and measure pH. • Prepare the client for x-ray checkup, if prescribed. *Comments:*	☐	☐	☐	
17. Connect the distal end of the tube to suction, draining bag, or adapter according to purpose of procedure. *Comments:*	☐	☐	☐	

continued on the following page

continued from the previous page

Procedure 31-1	**Able to Perform**	**Able to Perform with Assistance**	**Unable to Perform**	**Initials and Date**
18. Secure the tube with tape or a rubber band and safety pin to the client's gown. *Comments:*	☐	☐	☐	
19. Remove protective equipment, dispose of used materials appropriately, and wash hands. *Comments:*	☐	☐	☐	
20. Position the client comfortably with the call light within reach. *Comments:*	☐	☐	☐	
21. Document procedure. *Comments:*	☐	☐	☐	
Maintaining a Nasogastric Tube				
22. Wash hands and don gloves. *Comments:*	☐	☐	☐	
23. Check tube placement (following the steps in Action 16) before instilling anything per NG tube or at least every 8 hours. *Comments:*	☐	☐	☐	
24. Assess for signs that the tube has become blocked. *Comments:*	☐	☐	☐	
25. Do not irrigate or rotate a tube that has been placed during gastric or esophageal surgery. *Comments:*	☐	☐	☐	
26. Provide oral hygiene and assist the client to clean nares daily. *Comments:*	☐	☐	☐	
27. Remove gloves, dispose of used materials appropriately, and wash hands. *Comments:*	☐	☐	☐	
Evaluation				
1. Client's nutritional status improves. *Comments:*	☐	☐	☐	

Procedure 31-1	Able to Perform	Able to Perform with Assistance	Unable to Perform	Initials and Date
2. Client's nutritional needs are met with the assistance of tube feeding. *Comments:*	☐	☐	☐	
3. Client maintains a patent airway. *Comments:*	☐	☐	☐	
4. Client does not have diarrhea caused by NG feeding. *Comments:*	☐	☐	☐	
5. Mouth mucous membranes remain moist and intact. *Comments:*	☐	☐	☐	
6. Client maintains a normal fluid volume. *Comments:*	☐	☐	☐	
7. Client's stomach decompressed and comfort level increases. *Comments:*	☐	☐	☐	

Checklist for Procedure 31-2   Performing Venipuncture (Blood Drawing)

Name _____ Date _____

School _____

Instructor _____

Course _____

Procedure 31-2 **Performing Venipuncture (Blood Drawing)**	**Able to Perform**	**Able to Perform with Assistance**	**Unable to Perform**	**Initials and Date**
Assessment				
1. Determine which tests are ordered and any special conditions for the collection or handling of the specimen. *Comments:*	☐	☐	☐	
2. Assess the integrity of the veins to be used in the procedure. Identify any conditions that may contraindicate venipuncture. *Comments:*	☐	☐	☐	
3. Review the client's medical history to determine if there are any expected complications from the venipuncture. *Comments:*	☐	☐	☐	
4. Determine the client's ability to cooperate with the procedure. *Comments:*	☐	☐	☐	
5. Review the physician's or qualified practitioner's order. Check for appropriateness and frequency of tests. *Comments:*	☐	☐	☐	
Planning/Expected Outcomes				
1. The puncture site will not continue to bleed or hematoma. *Comments:*	☐	☐	☐	
2. The puncture site will show no evidence of infection. *Comments:*	☐	☐	☐	
3. The laboratory specimen will be properly acquired and appropriately handled after collection. *Comments:*	☐	☐	☐	
4. The client will understand the test's purpose and the procedure. *Comments:*	☐	☐	☐	

continued on the following page

continued from the previous page

Procedure 31-2	Able to Perform	Able to Perform with Assistance	Unable to Perform	Initials and Date
5. The client will report minimal anxiety from the procedure. *Comments:*	☐	☐	☐	
Implementation				
1. Check client's identification band and explain procedure before beginning. Wash hands. *Comments:*	☐	☐	☐	
2. Bring equipment to bedside, or client exam room. *Comments:*	☐	☐	☐	
3. Close curtain or door. *Comments:*	☐	☐	☐	
4. Raise or lower bed/table to a comfortable working height. *Comments:*	☐	☐	☐	
5. Assess extremities for the presence of an arteriovenous shunt used for dialysis or history of mastectomy. *Comments:*	☐	☐	☐	
6. Position the client's arm; extend arm to form straight line from shoulder to wrist. Place pillow or towel under upper arm to enhance extension. Client should be in a supine or semi-Fowler's position. *Comments:*	☐	☐	☐	
7. Apply disposable gloves. *Comments:*	☐	☐	☐	
8. Apply the tourniquet 3–4 inches above the venipuncture site. *Comments:*	☐	☐	☐	
9. Check for the distal pulse. *Comments:*	☐	☐	☐	
10. Have the client open and close fist several times, leaving fist clenched prior to venipuncture. *Comments:*	☐	☐	☐	
11. Maintain tourniquet for only 1–2 minutes. *Comments:*	☐	☐	☐	

Procedure 31-2	Able to Perform	Able to Perform with Assistance	Unable to Perform	Initials and Date
12. Identify the best venipuncture site through palpation. *Comments:*	☐	☐	☐	
13. Select the vein for venipuncture. *Comments:*	☐	☐	☐	
14. Prepare to obtain the blood sample: • Syringe method: Have appropriate-sized syringe and needle. • Vacutainer method: Attach double-ended needle to Vacutainer tube with the blood specimen tube resting inside the Vacutainer, without puncturing the stopper. *Comments:*	☐	☐	☐	
15. Cleanse the site according to agency protocol using a circular motion extending 2 inches beyond site. Allow to dry. *Comments:*	☐	☐	☐	
16. Remove the needle cover and warn that client will feel needlestick. *Comments:*	☐	☐	☐	
17. Pull the skin taut below the site. *Comments:*	☐	☐	☐	
18. Hold the needle or Vacutainer at 15- to 30-degree angle to the skin with the bevel up. *Comments:*	☐	☐	☐	
19. Slowly insert needle/Vacutainer. *Comments:*	☐	☐	☐	
20. Technique varies depending on equipment used: • Syringe method: Gently pull back on syringe plunger and look for blood return. Obtain desired amount of blood. • Vacutainer method: Advance specimen tube onto double-ended needle. After the tube is full of blood, grasp the holder firmly, remove the tube, and insert additional tubes as indicated. *Comments:*	☐	☐	☐	
21. After the specimen collection is completed, release the tourniquet. *Comments:*	☐	☐	☐	

continued on the following page

continued from the previous page

Procedure 31-2	Able to Perform	Able to Perform with Assistance	Unable to Perform	Initials and Date
22. Place gauze over the puncture site, without pressure, and withdraw the needle from the vein. *Comments:*	☐	☐	☐	
23. Apply pressure over the venipuncture site 2–3 minutes or until the bleeding has stopped. Tape the gauze or a Band-Aid over the site. *Comments:*	☐	☐	☐	
24. Syringe method: • Insert the syringe needle into the appropriate collection tubes and allow to fill. • You may also remove stopper from Vacutainer collection tube, remove needle from syringe, and fill tube. *Comments:*	☐	☐	☐	
25. Gently rotate tubes with additives 8–10 times. *Comments:*	☐	☐	☐	
26. Inspect the puncture site for bleeding. Reapply gauze and tape, if necessary. *Comments:*	☐	☐	☐	
27. Position client for comfort. Return bed to low position with side rails up, if appropriate. *Comments:*	☐	☐	☐	
28. Check tubes for external blood and decontaminate as appropriate. *Comments:*	☐	☐	☐	
29. Check tubes for proper labeling and packaging for transport to laboratory. *Comments:*	☐	☐	☐	
30. Dispose of needles, syringes, and soiled equipment appropriately. *Comments:*	☐	☐	☐	
31. Remove and dispose of gloves. *Comments:*	☐	☐	☐	

Procedure 31-2	Able to Perform	Able to Perform with Assistance	Unable to Perform	Initials and Date
32. Wash hands. *Comments:*	☐	☐	☐	
33. Send specimens to the laboratory. *Comments:*	☐	☐	☐	
Evaluation				
1. Venipuncture site shows no evidence of continued bleeding or hematoma. *Comments:*	☐	☐	☐	
2. Venipuncture site shows no signs or symptoms of infection. *Comments:*	☐	☐	☐	
3. Blood specimen is properly acquired and appropriately handled after collection. *Comments:*	☐	☐	☐	
4. Client is able to discuss the purpose of the test and describe the procedure. *Comments:*	☐	☐	☐	
5. Client reported minimal anxiety. *Comments:*	☐	☐	☐	

Checklist for Procedure 31-3   Preparing an IV Solution and Starting an IV

Name _____ Date _____

School _____

Instructor _____

Course _____

Procedure 31-3 **Preparing an IV Solution and Starting an IV**	Able to Perform	Able to Perform with Assistance	Unable to Perform	Initials and Date
Assessment				
1. Check the health care provider's order for the type of IV solution to be infused and the rate of flow. *Comments:*	☐	☐	☐	
2. Review information regarding the solution and insertion of the IV and nursing implications. *Comments:*	☐	☐	☐	
3. Know the agency's policy regarding who may start an IV. *Comments:*	☐	☐	☐	
4. Check all additives in the solution and other medications. *Comments:*	☐	☐	☐	
5. Assess the client's veins. *Comments:*	☐	☐	☐	
6. Check the client's fluid, electrolyte, and nutritional status. *Comments:*	☐	☐	☐	
7. Assess the client's understanding of the purpose of the procedure. *Comments:*	☐	☐	☐	
Planning/Expected Outcomes				
1. The appropriate fluids at the ordered dosages will be available for IV infusion. *Comments:*	☐	☐	☐	
2. The IV infusion will be sterile, without precipitate or contamination. *Comments:*	☐	☐	☐	
3. The IV will be inserted into the vein without complications and will remain patent. *Comments:*	☐	☐	☐	

continued on the following page

continued from the previous page

Procedure 31-3	Able to Perform	Able to Perform with Assistance	Unable to Perform	Initials and Date
4. Fluid and electrolyte balance will be restored. *Comments:*	☐	☐	☐	
5. Nutrition will be restored or maintained. *Comments:*	☐	☐	☐	
6. The IV site will remain free of swelling and inflammation. *Comments:*	☐	☐	☐	
Implementation				
1. Check health care provider's order for an IV and the solution. Identify client. *Comments:*	☐	☐	☐	
2. Wash hands. *Comments:*	☐	☐	☐	
3. Remove protective cover from solution bag. *Comments:*	☐	☐	☐	
4. Inspect the bag for leaks, tears, or cracks. Inspect the fluid for clarity, particulate matter, and color. Check expiration date. *Comments:*	☐	☐	☐	
5. Prepare a label for the IV bag: • Note date, time, and your initials. • Attach the label upside-down to the bag. *Comments:*	☐	☐	☐	
6. Open new infusion set. Unroll tubing and close roller clamp. *Comments:*	☐	☐	☐	
7. Remove the plastic tab covering the port and insert the full length of the spike into the bag's port. *Comments:*	☐	☐	☐	
8. Compress the drip chamber to fill halfway. *Comments:*	☐	☐	☐	
9. Loosen protective cap from end of tubing, open the roller clamp, and flush tubing with IV solution. *Comments:*	☐	☐	☐	

Procedure 31-3	Able to Perform	Able to Perform with Assistance	Unable to Perform	Initials and Date
10. Close the roller clamp and tighten the cap protector. *Comments:*	☐	☐	☐	
11. Take prepared fluid and needed equipment to bedside. *Comments:*	☐	☐	☐	
12. Check client's identification band and explain procedure before beginning. *Comments:*	☐	☐	☐	
13. Wash hands and put on mask and gown if needed. *Comments:*	☐	☐	☐	
14. Assess the extremities for the presence of an arteriovenous shunt used for dialysis or history of mastectomy before selecting an appropriate site for the IV. *Comments:*	☐	☐	☐	
15. Inspect potential sites: • Place a tourniquet around the upper arm. • Examine the veins as they dilate. • Palpate the vein to test for firmness. • Release the tourniquet. *Comments:*	☐	☐	☐	
16. Select vein for venipuncture. • Use most distal part of the vein first. • Avoid bony prominences, wrist or hand, dominant hand and arm, extremities with decreased sensation, and areas of skin affected by rash or infection. *Comments:*	☐	☐	☐	
17. Select appropriate IV needle or catheter. *Comments:*	☐	☐	☐	
18. Prepare supplies: • Place towel or drape on table and place supplies on field. • Open needle adapter end of IV tubing set. *Comments:*	☐	☐	☐	
19. Clip hair on skin at site, if necessary. *Comments:*	☐	☐	☐	

continued on the following page

continued from the previous page

Procedure 31-3	Able to Perform	Able to Perform with Assistance	Unable to Perform	Initials and Date
20. Ask the client to rest arm in a dependent position, if possible. *Comments:*	☐	☐	☐	
21. Put on disposable gloves. *Comments:*	☐	☐	☐	
22. Prepare insertion site: • Place absorbent drape under the arm. • Scrub the insertion site with three alcohol swabs, then three povidone-iodine swabs. (Note: Some facilities do not use povidone-iodine swabs. Follow facility protocol.) • Allow the povidone-iodine to dry. *Comments:*	☐	☐	☐	
23. Apply tourniquet 5–6 inches above the insertion site: • Secure tightly enough to occlude venous, not arterial, flow. • Check presence of distal pulse. *Comments:*	☐	☐	☐	
24. Perform the venipuncture: • Anchor the vein by stretching the skin against the direction of insertion 2–3 inches distal to the site. • Insert the stylet needle at a 10- to 30-degree angle, bevel up. • Watch for blood return in the flashback chamber. • Verify needle placement in a vein, not artery. • Advance one and one-quarter inch into the vein while it is parallel to the skin. • Loosen stylet and advance catheter into vein until the hub rests at the site. • Do not reinsert stylet. • Hold thumb over vein above catheter tip. • Release the tourniquet. *Comments:*	☐	☐	☐	
25. Attach IV tubing to ONC. • Stabilize the catheter with one hand. • Remove the stylet from ONC, or if using a safety catheter, push the button on the protective casing and stylet will fully retract into the casing. • Quickly release pressure over vein and quickly connect needle adapter of IV set to hub of ONC. • Begin infusion at slow rate to keep vein open. *Comments:*	☐	☐	☐	

Procedure 31-3	Able to Perform	Able to Perform with Assistance	Unable to Perform	Initials and Date
26. Secure catheter in place: • Place tape over the hub of the catheter. • Place transparent dressing over insertion site. • Secure tubing in loop fashion with tape. *Comments:*	☐	☐	☐	
27. Regulate the flow, or attach tubing to infusion device or rate controller if used. Turn on pump and set flow rate. *Comments:*	☐	☐	☐	
28. Remove gloves and dispose with all used materials. *Comments:*	☐	☐	☐	
29. Label dressing with date, time, size, and gauge of catheter. Follow protocol for scheduled dressing changes. *Comments:*	☐	☐	☐	
30. Wash hands. *Comments:*	☐	☐	☐	
Evaluation				
1. The appropriate fluids at the ordered dosages were available for IV infusion. *Comments:*	☐	☐	☐	
2. IV infusion was sterile, without precipitate or contamination. *Comments:*	☐	☐	☐	
3. IV was inserted into the vein without complications and remains patent. *Comments:*	☐	☐	☐	
4. Fluid and electrolyte balance were restored. *Comments:*	☐	☐	☐	
5. Nutrition was restored or maintained. *Comments:*	☐	☐	☐	
6. IV site remains free of swelling and inflammation. *Comments:*	☐	☐	☐	

Checklist for Procedure 31-4   Setting the IV Flow Rate

Name _____ Date _____

School _____

Instructor _____

Course _____

Procedure 31-4 Setting the IV Flow Rate	Able to Perform	Able to Perform with Assistance	Unable to Perform	Initials and Date
Assessment				
1. Check health care provider's order for the IV to be infused and the flow rate. Comments:	☐	☐	☐	
2. Review information regarding the solution and nursing implications. Comments:	☐	☐	☐	
3. Assess the patency of the IV. Comments:	☐	☐	☐	
4. Assess the skin at the IV site. Comments:	☐	☐	☐	
5. Assess the client's understanding of the purpose of the IV infusion. Comments:	☐	☐	☐	
Planning/Expected Outcomes				
1. The fluid will be infused into the vein without complications. Comments:	☐	☐	☐	
2. The IV catheter will remain patent. Comments:	☐	☐	☐	
3. The fluid and electrolyte balance will return to normal. Comments:	☐	☐	☐	
4. The client will be able to discuss the purpose of the IV therapy. Comments:	☐	☐	☐	

continued on the following page

continued from the previous page

Procedure 31-4	Able to Perform	Able to Perform with Assistance	Unable to Perform	Initials and Date
Implementation				
1. Check client's identification band and explain procedure before beginning. Check health care provider's order for the IV solution and rate of infusion. *Comments:*	☐	☐	☐	
2. Wash hands. *Comments:*	☐	☐	☐	
3. Prepare to set flow rate: • Have paper and pencil ready to calculate flow rate. • Review calibration in drops per milliliter (gtt/mL) of each infusion set. *Comments:*	☐	☐	☐	
4. Determine hourly rate by dividing total volume by total hours. *Comments:*	☐	☐	☐	
5. Mark a length of tape placed on the IV bag with the hourly time periods according to the rate. *Comments:*	☐	☐	☐	
6. Calculate the minute rate based on the drop factor of the infusion set. *Comments:*	☐	☐	☐	
7. Set flow rate: • Regular tubing; no device: Count drops in drip chamber for 1 minute while watching second hand of watch and adjust the roller clamp. • Infusion pump: Insert the tubing into the flow control chamber, select the rate, open the roller clamp, and push the start button. • Controller: Place IV bag 36 inches above the IV site, select the desired drops per minute, open the roller clamp, and count drops for 1 minute to verify the rate. • Volume control device: Place device between IV bag and insertion spike of IV tubing, fill with 1–2 hours of IV fluid, and count drops for 1 minute. *Comments:*	☐	☐	☐	
8. Monitor infusion rate and IV site for infiltration. *Comments:*	☐	☐	☐	

Procedure 31-4	Able to Perform	Able to Perform with Assistance	Unable to Perform	Initials and Date
9. Assess infusion when alarm sounds. *Comments:*	☐	☐	☐	
10. Wash hands. *Comments:*	☐	☐	☐	
Evaluation				
1. Fluid is infusing into the vein without complications. *Comments:*	☐	☐	☐	
2. IV catheter remains patent. *Comments:*	☐	☐	☐	
3. Fluid and electrolyte balance returned to normal. *Comments:*	☐	☐	☐	
4. Client is able to discuss the purpose of IV therapy. *Comments:*	☐	☐	☐	
5. Client receives the correct amount of IV fluid. *Comments:*	☐	☐	☐	

Checklist for Procedure 31-5   Administering Medications via Secondary Administration Sets (Piggyback)

Name _____ Date _____

School _____

Instructor _____

Course _____

Procedure 31-5 Administering Medications via Secondary Administration Sets (Piggyback)	Able to Perform	Able to Perform with Assistance	Unable to Perform	Initials and Date
Assessment				
1. Check health care provider's order or the medication administration record for the medication, dosage, time, and route of administration. *Comments:*	☐	☐	☐	
2. Review information regarding the drug. *Comments:*	☐	☐	☐	
3. Determine the additives in the solution of an existing IV line. *Comments:*	☐	☐	☐	
4. Assess the placement of the IV catheter in the vein. *Comments:*	☐	☐	☐	
5. Assess the skin at the IV site. *Comments:*	☐	☐	☐	
6. Check the client's drug allergy history. *Comments:*	☐	☐	☐	
7. Assess the client's understanding of the purpose of the medication. *Comments:*	☐	☐	☐	
8. Assess the compatibility of the piggyback IV medication with the primary IV solution. *Comments:*	☐	☐	☐	
Planning/Expected Outcomes				
1. The drug will be infused into the vein without complications. *Comments:*	☐	☐	☐	
2. The IV site will remain free of swelling and inflammation. *Comments:*	☐	☐	☐	

continued on the following page

continued from the previous page

Procedure 31-5	Able to Perform	Able to Perform with Assistance	Unable to Perform	Initials and Date
3. The client will be able to discuss the purpose of the drug. *Comments:*	☐	☐	☐	
4. The client is free from allergic reaction. *Comments:*	☐	☐	☐	
Implementation				
1. Check health care provider's order. *Comments:*	☐	☐	☐	
2. Wash hands. *Comments:*	☐	☐	☐	
3. Check client's identification arm band and explain procedure. *Comments:*	☐	☐	☐	
4. Prepare medication bag: • Close clamp on tubing of secondary infusion set. • Spike medication bag with secondary infusion tubing. • Open clamp. • Allow tubing to fill with solution. *Comments:*	☐	☐	☐	
5. Hang piggyback medication bag above level of primary IV bag. Use extender to lower the primary bag. *Comments:*	☐	☐	☐	
6. Connect piggyback tubing to primary tubing at Y-port: • For needleless system, remove port cap and connect tubing. • If a needle is used, clean port with antiseptic swab and insert small-gauge needle into center of port. • Secure tubing with adhesive tape. *Comments:*	☐	☐	☐	
7. Administer the medication: • Check the prescribed length of time for the infusion. • Regulate the flow rate of the piggyback by adjusting regulator clamp. • Observe that primary infusion has stopped during drug administration. *Comments:*	☐	☐	☐	

continued from the previous page

Procedure 31-5	Able to Perform	Able to Perform with Assistance	Unable to Perform	Initials and Date
8. Check primary infusion line when medication is finished: • Regulate primary infusion rate. • Leave secondary bag and tubing in place. *Comments:*	☐	☐	☐	
9. Dispose of all used materials and place needles in sharps container. *Comments:*	☐	☐	☐	
10. Wash hands. *Comments:*	☐	☐	☐	
Evaluation				
1. Drug was infused into the vein without complications. *Comments:*	☐	☐	☐	
2. IV site remained free of swelling and inflammation. *Comments:*	☐	☐	☐	
3. Client was able to discuss the purpose of the drug. *Comments:*	☐	☐	☐	

Checklist for Procedure 31-6   Assessing and Maintaining an IV Insertion Site

Name _____ Date _____

School _____

Instructor _____

Course _____

Procedure 31-6 **Assessing and Maintaining an IV Insertion Site**	Able to Perform	Able to Perform with Assistance	Unable to Perform	Initials and Date
Assessment				
1. Review the order for IV therapy. *Comments:*	☐	☐	☐	
2. Identify potential risk factors for fluid and electrolyte imbalances. *Comments:*	☐	☐	☐	
3. Assess for dehydration. *Comments:*	☐	☐	☐	
4. Assess for fluid overload. *Comments:*	☐	☐	☐	
5. Determine the client's risk for complications from IV therapy. *Comments:*	☐	☐	☐	
6. Observe IV site for complications. *Comments:*	☐	☐	☐	
7. Observe IV site for patency. *Comments:*	☐	☐	☐	
8. Assess the client's knowledge regarding the need for IV therapy. *Comments:*	☐	☐	☐	
Planning/Expected Outcomes				
1. The IV will remain patent, without infection or inflammation. *Comments:*	☐	☐	☐	
2. The fluid and electrolyte imbalance will return to and remain normal and will be maintained. *Comments:*	☐	☐	☐	

continued on the following page

continued from the previous page

Procedure 31-6	Able to Perform	Able to Perform with Assistance	Unable to Perform	Initials and Date
3. The client will be able to report signs of inflammation or infiltration. *Comments:*	☐	☐	☐	
4. The client's IV will be administered and maintained per order. *Comments:*	☐	☐	☐	
5. The client's IV dressing will remain intact, clean, and dry. *Comments:*	☐	☐	☐	

Implementation

	Able to Perform	Able to Perform with Assistance	Unable to Perform	Initials and Date
1. Check client's identification band and explain procedure before beginning. Review the health care provider's order for IV therapy. *Comments:*	☐	☐	☐	
2. Review the client's history for medical conditions or allergies. *Comments:*	☐	☐	☐	
3. Review the client's IV site record and intake and output record. *Comments:*	☐	☐	☐	
4. Wash hands. *Comments:*	☐	☐	☐	
5. Obtain the client's vital signs. *Comments:*	☐	☐	☐	
6. Check IV for correct fluid, additives, rate, and volume at the beginning of your shift. *Comments:*	☐	☐	☐	
7. Check IV tubing for tight connections every 4 hours. *Comments:*	☐	☐	☐	
8. Check gauze IV dressing hourly to be sure it is dry and intact. *Comments:*	☐	☐	☐	

Procedure 31-6	Able to Perform	Able to Perform with Assistance	Unable to Perform	Initials and Date
9. If gauze is not dry and intact, remove the dressing and observe site for redness, swelling, or drainage. *Comments:*	☐	☐	☐	
10. Replace with new dry gauze dressing if no problems noted at site. *Comments:*	☐	☐	☐	
11. If an occlusive dressing is used, do not remove dressing when assessing the site. *Comments:*	☐	☐	☐	
12. Observe vein track for redness, swelling, warmth, or pain hourly. *Comments:*	☐	☐	☐	
13. Document IV site findings on appropriate electronic medical record or IV flow sheet. *Comments:*	☐	☐	☐	
14. Wash hands. *Comments:*	☐	☐	☐	
Evaluation				
1. IV site is without complications of phlebitis and infiltration. *Comments:*	☐	☐	☐	
2. Client reported no signs or symptoms of redness, swelling, or pain. *Comments:*	☐	☐	☐	

Checklist for Procedure 31-7   Changing Central Venous Dressing

Name _____   Date _____

School _____

Instructor _____

Course _____

Procedure 31-7 **Changing Central Venous Dressing**	Able to Perform	Able to Perform with Assistance	Unable to Perform	Initials and Date
Assessment				
1. Assess the need for dressing change by noting the last dressing change documented in the medical record and standard care recommended by the manufacturer and the institution. *Comments:*	☐	☐	☐	
2. Assess the timing of the dressing change as it relates to medication, IV fluid and transfusion schedules, as well as the time of the client's daily shower or bath. *Comments:*	☐	☐	☐	
3. Assess the type of central venous access in place. *Comments:*	☐	☐	☐	
4. Assess the integrity of the skin at the site. *Comments:*	☐	☐	☐	
5. Asses the client's and caregiver's knowledge of the purpose and care of the catheter. *Comments:*	☐	☐	☐	
Planning/Expected Outcomes				
1. Client's skin is intact at catheter site, has normal color, is not edematous, and has no drainage. *Comments:*	☐	☐	☐	
2. Client has no signs of systemic infection. *Comments:*	☐	☐	☐	
3. Catheter and tubing are intact. *Comments:*	☐	☐	☐	
4. Client and caregiver are able to perform skin care and dressing change. *Comments:*	☐	☐	☐	

continued on the following page

continued from the previous page

Procedure 31-7	Able to Perform	Able to Perform with Assistance	Unable to Perform	Initials and Date
Implementation				
1. Check client's identification band and explain procedure before beginning. Wash hands. *Comments:*	☐	☐	☐	
2. Put on mask and gloves. *Comments:*	☐	☐	☐	
3. Remove old dressing. Do not dislodge central catheter. *Comments:*	☐	☐	☐	
4. Note drainage on dressing. *Comments:*	☐	☐	☐	
5. Inspect skin at insertion site for redness, tenderness, or swelling. *Comments:*	☐	☐	☐	
6. Palpate tunneled catheter for presence of Dacron cuff, using care not to palpate close to exit site. *Comments:*	☐	☐	☐	
7. Visually inspect catheter from hub to skin. *Comments:*	☐	☐	☐	
8. Remove gloves and don sterile gloves. *Comments:*	☐	☐	☐	
9. Clean exit site according to institutional protocol. Use alcohol wipes first, then povidone-iodine ointment swab beginning at the catheter and moving out in a circular manner for 3 cm to maintain aseptic technique. *Comments:*	☐	☐	☐	
10. Use povidone-iodine ointment to exit site if agency policy. *Comments:*	☐	☐	☐	
11. Apply transparent dressing. (Use gauze dressing if agency policy.) *Comments:*	☐	☐	☐	

continued from the previous page

Procedure 31-7	Able to Perform	Able to Perform with Assistance	Unable to Perform	Initials and Date
12. Label with date and time of dressing change. *Comments:*	☐	☐	☐	
13. Secure tubing to client's clothing. *Comments:*	☐	☐	☐	
14. Remove gloves and dispose of all used materials according to agency policy *Comments:*	☐	☐	☐	
15. Wash hands. *Comments:*	☐	☐	☐	
Evaluation				
1. Client's skin is intact at catheter site, has normal color, and is not edematous. *Comments:*	☐	☐	☐	
2. Client has no signs of systemic infection such as fever or malaise. *Comments:*	☐	☐	☐	
3. The central venous catheter and tubing are intact. *Comments:*	☐	☐	☐	
4. Client and caregiver are able to perform skin care and dressing change. *Comments:*	☐	☐	☐	

Checklist for Procedure 31-8   Removing Skin Sutures and Staples

Name _____ Date _____

School _____

Instructor _____

Course _____

Procedure 31-8 Removing Skin Sutures and Staples	Able to Perform	Able to Perform with Assistance	Unable to Perform	Initials and Date
Assessment				
1. Assess the wound. *Comments:*	☐	☐	☐	
2. Assess for any signs of infection. *Comments:*	☐	☐	☐	
3. Assess for any conditions that impede the healing process. *Comments:*	☐	☐	☐	
Planning/Expected Outcomes				
1. The wound is healing, with the edges well approximated. *Comments:*	☐	☐	☐	
2. There is no redness or signs of infection. *Comments:*	☐	☐	☐	
3. The procedure is performed with a minimum of pain and trauma to the client. *Comments:*	☐	☐	☐	
Implementation				
1. Check client's identification band and explain procedure before beginning. Wash hands. *Comments:*	☐	☐	☐	
2. Assess the wound to determine whether the edges of the wound are well-approximated and healing has occurred. *Comments:*	☐	☐	☐	
3. Close the door and curtains around the client's bed. *Comments:*	☐	☐	☐	

continued on the following page

continued from the previous page

Procedure 31-8	Able to Perform	Able to Perform with Assistance	Unable to Perform	Initials and Date
4. Raise the bed to a comfortable level. *Comments:*	☐	☐	☐	
5. Position the client for comfort with easy access and visibility to the suture line. *Comments:*	☐	☐	☐	
6. Drape the client so that only the suture area is exposed. *Comments:*	☐	☐	☐	
7. Open the suture removal kit and assemble supplies within easy access. *Comments:*	☐	☐	☐	
8. Apply clean gloves; remove old dressing and dispose of appropriately. *Comments:*	☐	☐	☐	
9. Remove gloves and wash hands. *Comments:*	☐	☐	☐	
10. If dressings are to be used, assemble equipment and supplies on sterile field. *Comments:*	☐	☐	☐	
11. • Apply sterile gloves. • Clean the incision with saline-soaked gauze, antiseptic swabs, or per institutional policy. *Comments:*	☐	☐	☐	
12. Removing an interrupted suture: • Use forceps to grasp the suture near the knot. *Comments:*	☐	☐	☐	
13. Place the curved edge of the scissors under the suture or near the knot. *Comments:*	☐	☐	☐	
14. Cut the suture close to the skin where the suture emerges from the skin. Pull the long end and remove in one piece. *Comments:*	☐	☐	☐	

Procedure 31-8	Able to Perform	Able to Perform with Assistance	Unable to Perform	Initials and Date
15. Removing a continuous suture: • Cut both the first and second suture before removing them. *Comments:*	☐	☐	☐	
16. Some policies require removal of every other suture, with removal of the remaining sutures to be done later. Assess the suture line to ensure that the edges remain approximated. *Comments:*	☐	☐	☐	
17. Discard removed sutures onto the gauze squares as they are removed. Dispose of gauze squares appropriately. *Comments:*	☐	☐	☐	
18. Assess the suture line to ensure that the edges remain approximated and that all sutures have been removed. *Comments:*	☐	☐	☐	
19. Apply adhesive strips or butterfly strips across the suture line to secure the edges. *Comments:*	☐	☐	☐	
20. Dispose of the soiled equipment. *Comments:*	☐	☐	☐	
21. Remove gloves and wash hands. *Comments:*	☐	☐	☐	
22. If removing staples: • Repeat Actions 2–11. • Use a staple extractor to remove every other staple. Place the lower tip of staple remover under the staple and squeeze the handles together. The ends of the staple will extract from the skin. • Move the staple away from the skin surface and release the staple into a disposal container. • Assess the wound for adherence. • Move on to the next staple if the skin has adhered well. • Repeat Actions 19–21. *Comments:*	☐	☐	☐	

continued on the following page

continued from the previous page

Procedure 31-8	Able to Perform	Able to Perform with Assistance	Unable to Perform	Initials and Date
Evaluation				
1. Wound is intact, edges are adhered, and there are no signs of infection or drainage. *Comments:*	☐	☐	☐	
2. Sutures/staples were removed with a minimum of pain and trauma to the client. *Comments:*	☐	☐	☐	